ALZHEIMER'S DISEASE —

HOW ITS BACTERIAL CAUSE WAS FOUND AND THEN DISCARDED

LAWRENCE BROXMEYER, MD

ISBN: 1491287357
ISBN 13: 9781491287354
Library of Congress Control Number: 2016906366
CreateSpace Independent Publishing Platform
North Charleston, South Carolina

For Stanley Chester, of the greatest generation—
an Alzheimer's victim

TABLE OF CONTENTS

INTRODUCTION

Der mentsh trakht un got lakht.
(Men think, and the Lord laughs.)
—*Yiddish Proverb*

Every seventy-two seconds, someone in America develops Alzheimer's disease (AD). And it has been said that almost everyone living long enough will eventually show evidence of Alzheimer's disease. Thus far, its cause has remained elusive.

Nevertheless, recently, study after study in which scientists have injected human Alzheimer-diseased brain tissue into mice and other laboratory animals that later developed the disease have left little doubt that Alzheimer's arises from an infectious process[1-3]—the focus of debate seeming to be which particular disease. But clearly, whatever the infectious cause behind Alzheimer's is, it must be a disease that is statistically widespread in the world today and that was also prevalent at the time of Dr. Alzheimer.

Yet in 1901, when physician/psychiatrist Alzheimer observed a fifty-one-year-old woman named Auguste Deter at the Community Frankfurt Psychiatric Hospital in Frankfurt-am-Main, the three most striking things about her were her severe weight loss, her strange behavioral/psychiatric symptoms, and her loss of memory laced with confusion. Auguste was married and had a normal life until eight months prior to her confinement. Along with difficulties with memory and language, she showed paranoia, disorientation, auditory hallucinations, and delusions. At times, Deter was so delirious and her "they're-out-to-get-me" paranoia so severe that it bounced around from occasionally thinking someone was trying to kill her — to an unfounded jealousy of her husband — to loudly protesting that Alzheimer himself was trying to operate on or at times molest her.[4]

This patient would become Alzheimer's obsession over the coming years. And when in April 1906 Frau Deter, age fifty-six, died, curled up in a fetal position in that same City Asylum in Frankfort, nicknamed "Irrenschloss" (Castle of the Insane), her chart seemed to contain an extensive psychiatric workup with little effort to rule out any possible infectious disease behind her early cachectic death. Soon thereafter, Alzheimer had her records and her autopsied brain brought to Munich, where he was working at psychiatrist Emil Kraepelin's lab. Oddly, in his own writings Alzheimer never identified himself first as the top-notch neuropathologist he was, but rather simply as a clinical psychiatrist responsible for patients. And the way in which he documented and diagnosed Deter's case in that chart was certainly how a clinical psychiatrist would go about doing things.

But in far-off Scotland, where he read about Deter, Sir Thomas Clouston could not in any way agree with Alzheimer's thoughts or conclusions. To Clouston, Deter represented neither a "new disease" nor what Alzheimer referred to as "a peculiar, little-known disease process." Clouston, a contemporary of Alzheimer, would die in 1915—eight months to the day before Alzheimer's death. Clouston wasn't just a psychiatrist; at the time he was superintendent of the prestigious Royal Edinburgh Asylum and previous to that, president of the Royal College of Physicians.

Both Alzheimer and Clouston would soon hold international reputations, each considered a pioneer in the treatment of mental illness. Yet for the life of him, Sir Thomas Smith Clouston thought the case of gaunt, suspicious, hallucinatory, paranoid-like Auguste Deter an open and shut case of what he often referred to in his lectures at Edinburgh University as "monomania of suspicion." Clouston said this:

> This is a good example of those cases of pure monomania of suspicion, almost all of whom, according to my statistics, die of tuberculosis.[5]

As for the more demented cases such as Deter's, with her incapacitating memory loss, Clouston added this statement:

> This happens in about 30% of cases. It is the event we most dread. It is the equivalent to a mental death.[5]

So common was the knowledge at Alzheimer's time that tuberculosis (TB), in any form, whether inside or outside of the central nervous system, could lead to memory loss—some of it severe and progressive—that Clouston was just amazed at the exquisite lengths and efforts that Alzheimer and his boss, Kraepelin, went to totally ignore it. The fact that central nervous system tuberculosis could masquerade as an age-related Alzheimer's dementia with severe memory loss was and still is documented to this day:[6]

> Clouston maintained that since tuberculosis's psychiatric symptoms and dementia appeared long before the disease itself advanced to any great degree, many

patients committed with TB were being sent to asylums instead of special hospitals for the treatment of the disease. Carpenter, in a 1903 review in *The Journal of the American Medical Association*, found Clouston's opinions not only justified but "a decisive etiologic [causative] factor" in any discussion of a subset of all asylum populations,[7] including the one Auguste Deter now found herself in. Forbes Winslow of Sussex House Hammersmith, himself a former president of the Royal College of Psychiatry prior to Clouston, had documented what neurotuberculosis could do to the mind in a clear and methodical way. Winslow presented cases[8] of severe mental loss at the hands of neurotuberculosis. Among them, a gentleman, aged fifty-four who worked as a principal in a fairly large school and who died of "softening of the brain," as his tubercular disease choked off vital blood supply to that portion of the brain. This man, who was Deter's age, had admitted at the time to his medical attendant that his mind was "gradually fading away from him," yet he carried on, occupying himself with his usual workday duties—until one day he could not. Winslow said this: "Immediately retiring to his own private room, he seated himself in a chair, burst into a flood of tears, exclaiming, in wild despair, 'My mind is gone! Altogether gone!'" [Ibid., p. 327]

In this case, no symptoms of physical [tubercular] disease of the brain were detected until twelve months before death. In another case, a retired army officer's mind appeared to gradually fade away and succumb to a mysterious influence. Only after death did the reason become apparent. The dura mater of his brain was riddled with tuberculosis, his brain much shrunken, and in some portions, was in a softened state. In this instance, there were no delusions or other symptoms of mental abnormality until a year and a half before death. Forbes Winslow was citing these kinds of cases, Clouston knew, to point out that structural disease of the brain from cerebral tuberculosis could occasionally be preceded by no other symptom than the loss of mental power and memory.

Clouston thought it odd, then, that in 1905, a year before Deter died, Paul Claisse and his colleague, Dr. Abrami, presented a case to the Medical Society of the Hospitals of Paris,[9] with much the same symptomatology of Frau Deter, both psychiatrically and neurologically. But in this case, a spinal tap was offered and performed, something which Deter's family was never afforded the opportunity of choosing. The spinal fluid drawn from this patient showed lymphocytosis (an increase in those white blood cells called lymphocytes). And when it was injected into a guinea pig, that guinea pig abruptly expired—of tuberculosis. Despite this, Claisse and Abrami's patient went on to make a satisfactory recovery.

In Alzheimer's time, there were two major and often deadly infectious diseases that filled nineteenth-century and early twentieth-century psychiatric asylums: tuberculosis and syphilis. Deter did not have syphilis. Alzheimer documented that Deter did not even have the "suggestion of" neurosyphilis.[17] But by measure of weight loss and Deter's skeletal emaciation alone, she obviously did have a chronic wasting disease. Although there are estimates in place that more than 25 percent of chronic psychiatric patients in asylums circa 1900 had neurosyphilis, by 1905—one year before Alzheimer presented his findings on Deter's brain to the Thirty-Seventh Meeting of Southwest German Psychiatrists at Tübingen—a German report[10] surfaced saying otherwise. It indicated that besides tubercular disease, the only two other truly statistically significant illnesses leading toward what could only be described as a nineteenth-century surge in psychiatric disease—neurosyphilis and alcoholism, combined—represented no more than a small statistical portion of asylum populations. Their incidence was 11 percent combined for the State of Prussia, largest within unified Germany, where Alzheimer worked for Kraepelin. This study was done based on new admissions to German asylums. Therefore, the overwhelming rate of tubercular admissions cited could not be attributed to "unsanitary asylum conditions" or to "overcrowding" once inside an asylum.

Tellingly, Alzheimer's original presentation of Auguste Deter's pathology at a November 1906 conference in Tubingen, Germany, was disappointing. The meeting's chairman, Alfred Hoche, despised Alzheimer's employer, Kraepelin. Hoche had little use for Kraepelin's ever-changing psychiatric classifications. Kraepelin, for his part, though absent from the meeting, had every intention of naming the disease that Alzheimer was presenting under what Hoche considered yet another unnecessary classification: Alzheimer's disease. If it were not for Hoche's animosity, Kraepelin would certainly have attended this meeting. And although Chairman Hoche and his German colleagues listened respectfully to Alzheimer, there were remarkably no questions after Alzheimer's talk. Seizing the opportunity, Hoche abruptly relieved Alzheimer of the podium. Other issues stirred much more interest and passion, such as whether Freud's concepts should be accepted:

> Alzheimer had opened his Deter presentation by saying this: "Clinical observation alone made the case appear so unusual that it could not be classified as one of the recognized illnesses; it showed anatomical characteristics which set it apart from all recognized cases."[4]

This wasn't entirely true. First, there was very little that set the anatomical characteristics of Alzheimer's findings apart from senile dementia. Second, by 1830, Papavoine[11] had already described "plaques" in the brain, associated with systemic tuberculosis present either in or outside the brain. And as for the location where Papavoine noticed such plaques, they were in the brain's pia mater, the innermost of the three coverings of the brain called the *meninges*. This was the very area in which neuropathologist Perusini,[12] who by 1910 was Alzheimer's go-to pathologist, showed alterations similar to Papavoine's pial changes in all four of his Alzheimer's autopsies. In addition, approximately ten years before Alzheimer wrote about Deter, Ludvig Hektoen, former editor of *The Journal of Infectious Diseases*, was already defining many of the same vascular changes in neurotuberculosis[13] of the brain that Alzheimer and Perusini now documented as an integral part of their "new" disease.

In fact, at the very time that Alzheimer autopsied Deter's brain, German investigators[14,15,16] were issuing voluminous literature defining a constellation of tubercular signs, symptoms, and tissue findings, many of which Deter actually had. These included failure of memory, auditory hallucinations, delusions, incoherence, delirium, loss of the ability to use words, incontinence, and hydrocephalus. Yet Alzheimer persisted in his seeming ostrich-like approach, burying his head in the sand, insisting on Alzheimer's disease as a "peculiar disease process [which has been] verified recently in large numbers." And this was a statement made at a time when tuberculosis's annual kill rate was an incredible seven million persons per year—threatening the very existence of civilized Europe. In response, Germany, with its back against the wall, facing a disease whose bacillus had been found but whose cure had not, began to churn out one TB sanatorium treatment center after another. And so it was, that as Alois Alzheimer pursued his clinical and laboratory duties, there was hardly a single large township or district in all of Germany that had not constructed its own open-air, hygienic-treatment tubercular sanatorium for its "consumptives."[17]

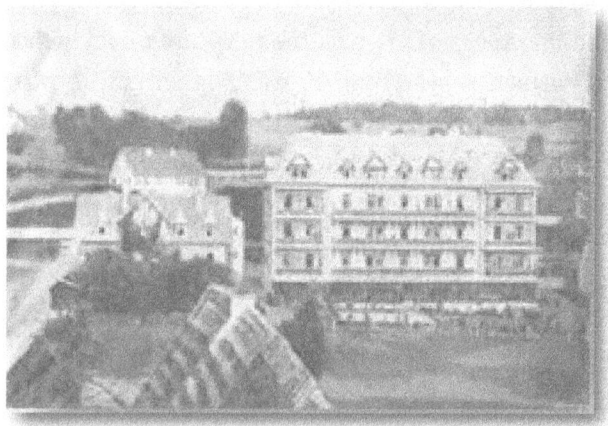

Figure 1. View of the Schomberg TB Sanatarium in Germany—one of many.

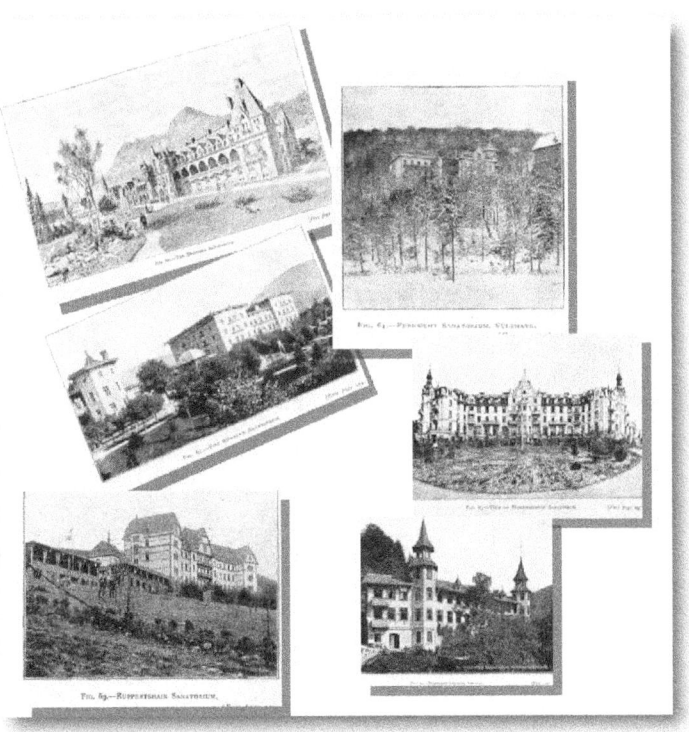

Figure 2. Some of the other fortress-like TB sanatoria dotting Germany circa Alzheimer's time.

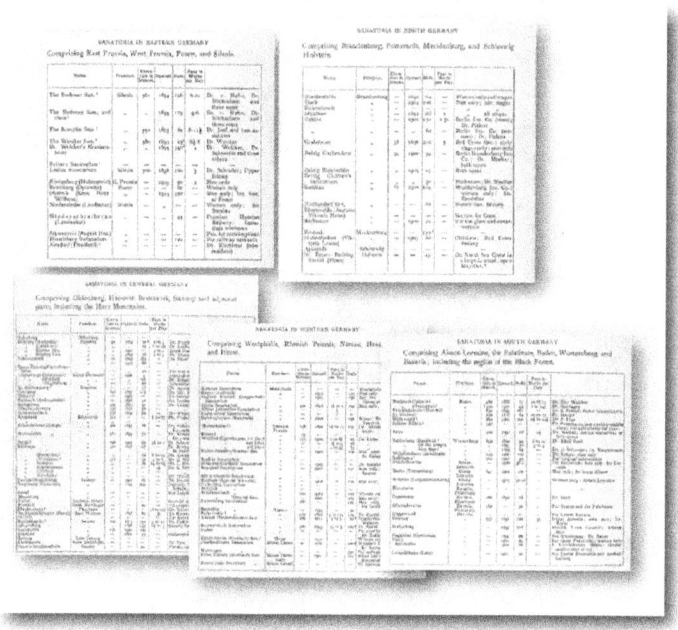

Figure 3. A more comprehensive list of the burgeoning, ever-growing German TB treatment sanatoria operative throughout unified Germany during Dr. Alzheimer's career (From F. R. Walters, Sanatoria for Consumptives, Swan Sonnenschein & Company, Ltd., London, 1899.)

Alzheimer would continue to speak about the pathology he had found in Alzheimer's disease: "Very remarkable and really without precedent in the pathological anatomy of the nervous system are the alterations of [brain neuron] axis-cylinders [the central core of the axon of in this case brain neurons], so exhaustively described by Fischer."[18]

But, in reality, again, nothing was mentioned without "precedent." True, Fischer, Alzheimer's great European rival, was credited with establishing senile dementia, which he felt was part and parcel of Alzheimer's disease and exhaustively worked on the alterations in axon cores in Alzheimer's. Yet Barlow,[18] in describing neurotuberculosis seven years prior to Alzheimer and Fischer's work, mentioned both Fischer's degenerative plaque alterations in the brain's neuronal axis-cylinders and Alzheimer's own observation with regard to the fibrillary degenerative tangles of cerebral ganglion cells under tubercular attack. Here is Barlow's explanation for such tuberculous "plaques" and "tangles":

> Microscopic investigations throws some light upon this condition [tubercular meningoencephalitis]: the deposition of miliary tubercle in the subarachnoid, and along the ingrowing processes of pia mater, not only interferes with the vascular nutrition of the brain substance, but actually invades it, giving rise to extensive cellular infiltration, and causing degeneration of both axis-cylinders [of brain neurons] and ganglion cells. This seems to justify the modern designation of the disease as a true [tubercular] meningoencephalitis.[19]

Barlow, who knew that tubercular meningoencephalitis was looked on, then as now, as almost invariably fatal, felt the need for clarification:

> Finally, it is to be noted that the supervening of tubercular meningitis on severe or extensive tuberculous disease elsewhere in the body is sometimes quite latent, and not discovered till after death.[19]

If statistically TB meningitis was being defined as the most common form of cerebral tuberculosis, it was simply because these were the cases that desperately sought medical attention and presented themselves at hospitals. But for a person to have meningitis, the disease had to break through to the spinal fluid, which in many cases never happened; and if it did, often it did so much later in the disease process. In the meantime, the spectrum of cerebral tuberculosis was much more extensive than TB meningitis, as witnessed by the not uncommon appearance of silent tubercles in the brain at autopsy. In his fifth edition of the *Pathologic Basis of Disease*, Robbins[20] used the term "diffuse chronic meningoencephalitis" as the most common pattern of tubercular involvement of the brain. He also acknowledged that its symptoms could vary greatly, ranging from simply chronic or intermittent headache with subtle mental changes to full-blown meningitis. As early as 1911, German physician/investigator Roepke, and Otto Ranke before him in 1908, emphasized that cerebral tuberculosis was not necessarily a death sentence and that often it was simply a matter of such small, multiple blood-borne tubercles landing in a particular area in the brain, usually early in life.

Arnold Rich, head of pathology at Johns Hopkins, would confirm this decades later.[21] In fact, to Rich, just if and where in the brain that bloodborne tuberculosis landed was tantamount to what card players call the "luck of the draw," with many brain tubercles, silent and quiescent, being picked up only by radiologic tests or at autopsy decades later. Ranke's article[16] is a careful report on the tissue pathology of neurotuberculosis, which should have been of interest to anyone pursuing the cause of Alzheimer's disease. Many of Otto Ranke's drawings in this paper, created with the Camera Lucida of that era, showed a decimation of cerebral nervous tissue similar to those drawn by Perusini and Alzheimer themselves.

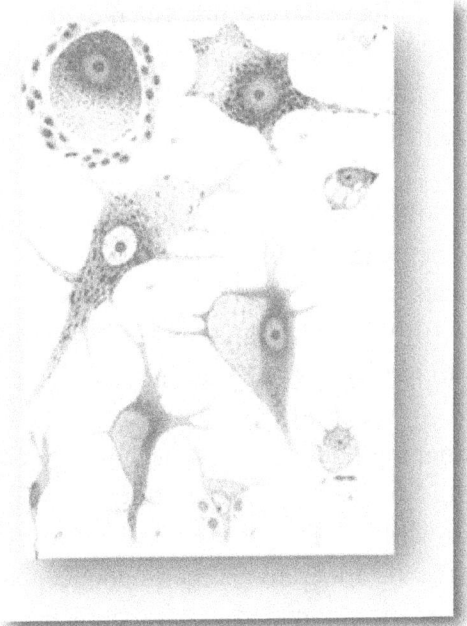

Figure 4. Some of Ranke's drawings depicting pathology in cerebral tuberculosis.

Ranke saw as the body's defenders against tubercular infection not only blood macrophages (a type of scavenger white blood cell) of varying morphology in pial blood vessels in the brain, but galvanized glial forms in the brain's parenchyma. The glia or microglia have long been called the macrophages of the brain, which, along with blood macrophages, attempt to stamp out and remove debris from, among other things, cerebral infection. However, in the case of an acute virulent tubercular meningeal assault, such an attempt was rarely successful. And what Ranke noticed instead was a markedly violent infection that seeped further into brain matter, leaving severely injured, shriveled, darkly stained pyknotic neurons and ganglion cells in its inflammatory path. Ranke also detected nerve and ganglion cells die off when they were under tubercular assault. Such neuronal death would soon be replaced by the same stop-gap clustered, proliferating glial forms mentioned by some in Alzheimer's group—with occasional rod cells.

It is improbable that Alois Alzheimer did not read and absorb the parallels between Ranke's work on central nervous system tuberculosis and his own histological findings on Auguste Deter's brain. In 1904, Alzheimer and his lifetime friend, Franz Nissl, began to jointly edit the journal *Histologische und histopathologische Arbeiten uber die Grosshirnrinde*—a publication Ranke's TB meningitis review was accepted into and then published in 1908. Ranke's paper also cited the experimental work of Kure, who, while working in Nissl's laboratory in 1898, produced experimental tuberculous meningoencephalitis by drawing cotton threads impregnated with tubercle bacilli through the brains of dogs.

Despite such knowledge of possible linkage between cerebral tuberculosis and Alzheimer's disease—an association implied not only by Alzheimer's German and European colleagues but subsequently by Southard at Harvard and Clouston at Edinburgh—and despite the seven million deaths per year from a tubercular disease that led to TB sanatoria sprouting up like weeds all around him—Alzheimer's silence was singular. Alzheimer doubled down on his carefully manicured hypothesis, repeatedly beseeching neurologists and psychiatrists alike not to look toward "well-known disease" as being behind this "new disease." After all, it had to be a "new" disease because Alzheimer's chief, Emil Kraepelin, demanded that it be new.

NOTES

1. H. F. Baker, R. M. Ridley, L. W. Duchen, T. J. Crow, and C. J. Bruton, "Induction of Beta (A4)-Amyloid in Primates by Injection of Alzheimer's Disease Brain Homogenate: Comparison with Transmission of Spongiform Encephalopathy," *Molecular Neurobiology* 8, no. 1 (February 1994): 25–39.

2. M. D. Kane, W. J. Lipinski, M. J. Callahan, F. Bian, R. A. Durham, R. D. Schwartz, A. E. Roher, and L. C. Walker, "Evidence for Seeding of ß-Amyloid by Intracerebral Infusion of Alzheimer Brain Extracts in ß-Amyloid Precursor Protein-Transgenic Mice.," *The Journal of Neuroscience* 20, no. 10 (May 15, 2000: 3606–11.

3. R. Morales, C. Duran-Aniotz, J. Castilla, L. D. Estrada, and C. Soto, "De Novo Induction of Amyloid-β Deposition in vivo. *Molecular Psychiatry* 17, no. 12 (December 2012):1347–53.

4. R. A. Stelzmann, H. N. Schnitzlein, and F. R. Murtagh, an English translation of Alzheimer's 1907 paper "Uber Eine Eigenartige Erkankung der Hirnrinde," *Clinical Anatomy* 8 (1995):429–31.

5. Clouston, TS. Illustrations of Phthisical Insanity. Journal of Mental Science 1864; 50:220-229, p. 210.

6. N. K. Sethi, P. K. Sethi, J. Torgovnick, and E. Arsura, "Central Nervous System Tuberculosis Masquerading as Primary Dementia: A Case Report," *Neurologia i Neurochirurgia Polska* 45, no. 5 (September–October 2011): 510–3.

7. E. G. Carpenter, "Determinate Factors in the Cause of Insanity," Journal of the American Medical Association 60, no. 4 (January1903): 240–4.

8. F. Winslow, *On Obscure Diseases of the Brain and Disorders of the Mind: Their Incipient Symptoms, Pathology, Diagnosis,*

Treatment, and Prophylaxis (London: John Churchill Publishers, April 1860).

9. P. Claisse and Abrami, "Un Cas de Méningite Tuberculeus Terrninee par Guerison," *Bull. et mém. soc. méd. d. hop. de Par.* 22 (1905):390–403.

10. H. Grunau, "Uber Frequenz, Heilerfolge, und Sterblichkeit in den Offentliochen preussischen Irrenanstalten von 1875 bis 1900 (Halle: Carl Marhold, 1905).

11. Louis-Nicolas Papavoine, "Propositions Sur les Tubercules Consideres Specialement Chez le Enfans," dissertation no. 86, v. 231 (Paris, 1830).

12. G. Perusini, *Histology and Clinical Findings of Some Psychiatric Diseases of Older People in Histologische und histopathologishe*, vol. III, edited by F. Arbeiten Nissl and A. Alzheimer, (Jena, Germany: Gustav Fischer, 1910), 297–351.

13. Ludvig Hektoen, "The Vascular Changes of Tuberculous Meningitis, Especially with Tuberculous Endarteritis," *The Journal of Experimental Medicine* 1, no. 112 (1896).

14. B. Bandelier and O. Roepke, *A Clinical System of Tuberculosis*, Translated from the Second German Edition by G. Band and Bertram Hunt, MD (New York: William Wood and Company 1913).

15. Bandelier R, Roepke O. *Lehrbuch der Spezifischen Diagnostic und Therapie der tuberkulose: Fur Arzte und Studierende* (Wurzburg : Curt Kabitzsch, 1911).

16. O. Ranke, *Beitrage zur Lehre von der Meningitis tuberculoa.* Edited by Franz Nissl and Alois Alzheimer; *Histologische und Histopathologische Arbeiten uber die Grosshirnrinde* (Jena, Germany: Verlag Von Gustave Fischer, 1908), 252–347.

17. F. R. Walters, *Sanatoria for Consumptives* (London: Swan Sonnenschein & Company, Ltd., 1899).

18. A. Alzheimer, "Uber Eigenartige Krankheitsfalle des Spateren Alters," *Zeitschrift fur die Gesamte Neurologie und Psychiatrie* 4 (1911): 356–85.
19. T. Barlow, *Tuberculous Meningitis in a System of Medicine by Many Writers*, edited by Thomas Clifford Allbutt, vol. vii (New York: The Macmillan Company, 1899): 466–91.
20. S. L. Robbins, *Robbins Pathologic Basis of Disease,* 5th ed. (Philadelphia: W. B. Saunders Company, 1994).
21. A. R. Rich, *The Pathogenesis of Tuberculosis* (Springfield, Illinois: Chas C. Thomas, 1946).

CHAPTER 1

Department of Neuropsychiatry, the German University of Prague, Prague, Czechoslovakia, 1907

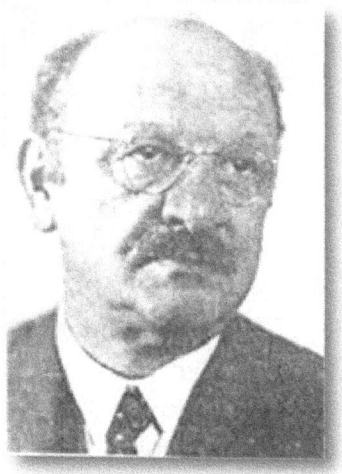

Figure 5. Alzheimer's great rival, Oskar Fischer (1876–1942), around the time of his sixtieth birthday in 1936.

It thus becomes a matter of great curiosity and interest that from the beginning, Alois Alzheimer's main rival, German neuro-pathologist Oskar Fischer, thought he had spotted, throughout his Alzheimer's brain autopsies, a tubercular-like germ called *Streptothrix*, often confused with the filamentous forms of the tubercular bacilli. For Fischer, this was the possible infectious cause of Alzheimer's.

Fischer's findings were never meant to be taken lightly. Historical circumstance mandates that we owe as much to Oskar Fischer for the discovery of Alzheimer's disease as to Alois Alzheimer himself. Doubters have to go no further than Alzheimer's 1911 paper,[1] which is in part a running dialogue between Alzheimer's own feelings and findings and those of the Prague Institute of Neurology's Dr. Oskar Fischer. Indeed, the only reason why what we call "Alzheimer's disease today is not called "Alzheimer–Fischer's disease" or just "Fischer's disease" has simply to do with the course of world history, the rise of Nazi Germany, and Alzheimer's boss, Emil Kraepelin, high priest of early German psychiatry.

A Prague neuropathologist of German–Jewish origin, for years Oskar Fischer's presbyophrenia—a form of senile dementia characterized by marked memory loss—and Alzheimer's disease, supposedly a "presenile" dementia, were used interchangeably. Yet even after Alzheimer's findings became known, Simchowitz, first to use the term "senile plaque," wrote in 1914 that there was no difference between Alzheimer's disease and Fischer's senile dementia.[2] And in a 1916 review, Spielmeyer, who would eventually replace Alzheimer at Munich, revealed that even Alzheimer himself knew that the presenile decline he had "discovered" in people in their late forties, fifties, and early sixties was nothing really new.[3] It was simply what Fischer had already characterized with somewhat of an earlier age of onset, at a time when certain pathologic findings were more prominent.

Fischer knew this, but it would take decades for others to confirm his thoughts with tissue studies.[4] At that point, rather than incorporate the disproven presenile "Alzheimer's disease" (AD) back into Fischer's senile dementia, quite the opposite occurred: the designation "Alzheimer's disease" assumed the mantle of both presenile and senile dementia,[5] a major reason for its inflated preeminence in today's disease hierarchy.

It has also become more and more obvious that just as Oskar Fischer implicated to begin with, there is an association between dementias such as Alzheimer's and infectious disease.[6,7] Often, Alzheimer's plaque looks like colonies of bacteria, which would account for the disease's chronic inflammation that damages brain neurons. But what has recently brought this microbial hypothesis into sharper focus than ever have been microscopic findings that microbes such as tuberculosis, a disease historically associated with human amyloidosis to begin with, can produce amyloid fibrils identical to those found in Alzheimer's plaque.[8] Moreover, such bacteria-manufactured amyloid fibrils elicit the same response from the brain's immune cells as does Alzheimer's amyloid plaque, the sticky buildup of proteins that accumulates outside of Alzheimer's nerve cells.[9] Kidd confirmed as early as 1963 that the amyloid of Alzheimer's was indistinguishable from amyloid generated by an infection such as TB.[10]

But to be sure, Oskar Fischer was the first on record to suggest that infection might be causative for either Alzheimer's presenile dementia or his own senile dementia.[11] Fischer's infectious view never gained immediate popularity, although today, more than a century later, a volume of data supporting such an approach has begun to accumulate. But was Fischer's specific microbe on the right track to discovering the cause of Alzheimer's to begin with? Documents uncovered since then seem to suggest that he was considerably closer than anyone else—either then or since.

But history was about to intervene. During a few of Fischer's most productive years in Prague, a young Albert Einstein worked just blocks from him. Einstein was among the established Jewish thinkers in science who got out of Europe before the Nazis could destroy them. Oskar Fischer, however—despite warning after warning—did not. First he lost his tenure and then his teaching privileges at Prague's Charles University. By 1939, the Nazis occupied Prague, and one of their first reprisals against Czech society was aimed at education. Prague's Charles University, already separated into Czech and German parts, was, by September 1, 1939, subordinated to the Reich Ministry of Education in Berlin and approximately two months later, proclaimed to be known as Reichsuniversitat. When this met with resistance, Nazi authorities closed down Charles altogether. This occurred on November 17, 1939, for what was supposed to be a period limited to three years. However, the Nazis never had any intention of allowing Charles to open again, and many of its professors and students were sent to their early camp deaths directly from that university.

That same year, Fischer was somehow able to open a private office for neurology and psychiatry in Prague. But within three years of the German invasion, he was arrested and promptly sent to the Nazi concentration camp at Terezin (Theresienstadt), set up in a garrison town near Prague. Oskar Fischer died there on February 28, 1942, allegedly from a heart attack. He was sixty-five. The Nazis had erased more than a man. They had almost blotted out an entire concept on Alzheimer's infectious origin. But Fischer's accomplishments would lay untouched in Czech archives, to be rediscovered one day, primarily by the investigative efforts of Dr. Michael Goedert.[12]

During this same time in the existence of the Third Reich, while Hitler was still in power, the three children who had survived Alois Alzheimer and his Jewish wife were cared for in a house just outside Munich. They survived simply because they were inoculated from certain death by being the children of Alois Alzheimer, who by that time was a celebrated German icon.

As a member of the Prague School of Neuropathology, headed by famed neuropathologist Arnold Pick, Oskar Fischer's credentials were flawless. At the time, the Prague school was one of two neuropathological schools in Europe. The other was in Munich, headed by Emil Kraepelin, where Alzheimer worked. Fischer's detailed drawings showed neuritic Alzheimer brain plaque with abnormal, club-shaped neurons (see fig. 6) and small branching complexes—leading to the displacement of the rest of the normal-looking nerve fibrils in the space occupied by the plaques. These where the "drüsen," occasionally club-shaped, that Fischer repeatedly wrote about.

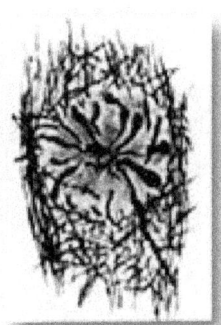

Figure 6. The thick, black, club-shaped "Drüsen" in Oskar Fischer's 1907 drawing of senile plaque.

At the time, it was widely acknowledged that such drüsen could result from either infection with *Streptothrix*, now known as actinomycosis (aktinomycesdruse), a rare disease in humans, or tuberculosis, a disease that by 1882, as Alzheimer prepared to leave for Berlin for his medical education, was understood to be far and away the leading cause of infectious death in Europe. During Alzheimer's and Fischer's lifetimes, tuberculosis's annual death rate of seven million persons per year was more than twice the approximately two million to three million people some estimate it still kills annually.[13] Furthermore, clinically there has always been a subset in adults with cerebral tuberculosis whose clinical features included a slowly progressive dementia over months or years characterized by, among other things, memory deficits.[14]

The disease actinomycosis was at one time referred to interchangeably with its older bacterial name, the *"Streptotriches"* (the plural form of *Streptothrix*). Fischer used such older nomenclature in describing certain forms he saw under his microscope.

Although Paul Oscar Blocq and Gheorghe Marinescu[15] had first described senile plaque fifteen years prior to Fischer, they failed to relate it to age-related dementia, nor were they willing to stipulate a possible bacteriological cause, as Fischer did. This omission of a potential cause was despite the uncanny resemblance between some of Marinescu's drawings[16] of senile plaque and Oskar Fischer's drüsen.

Tubercular cerebral plaque, one subset of which is called *tuberculoma en plaque,* was first described by French authors, notably

Chantemesse[17] in 1884, eight years before Blocq and Marinescu stumbled across their "senile" plaque.

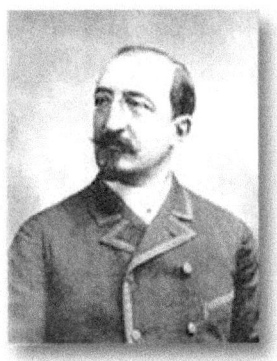

Figure 7. Andre Chantemesse (1851–1919).

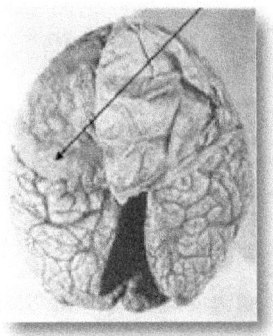

Figure 8. A case of tuberculoma en plaque. The brain's covering (dura) has been reflected back from the left frontal cortex to show the cortical plaque from tuberculosis (see arrow).

Chantemesse's cerebral plaque was a chronic, proliferating, fibroid type of tuberculosis, with extensive areas involving the meninges of the brain's cortex. The average survival with such tubercular plaque-ridden brain disease was approximately seven years. Most people who have Alzheimer's disease die within eight years of their diagnosis—typically from infection or "pneumonia," not cognitive failure.

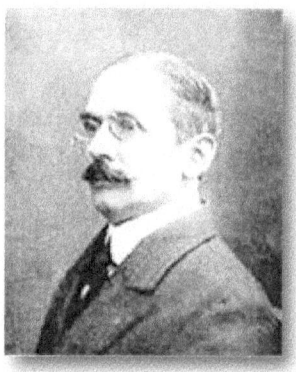

Figure 9. Physician and early bacteriologist Victor Babes (1854–1926). He made significant contributions to the study of rabies, diphtheria, tuberculosis, and other infectious diseases. Gheorghe Marinescu began his career as Babes's assistant. It is Babes who got Marinescu a scholarship, allowing him to spend nine years in Paris studying neurology under Charcot.

Victor Babes might have been among the first bacteriologists, but he also had a sharp interest in the nervous system. Later he, Blocq, and Marinescu would publish *An Atlas of the Pathologic Histology of the Nervous System*.[18]

Neither Blocq, Marinescu, nor Oskar Fischer were bacteriologists, but Victor Babes was. Born in Vienna, Babes at one point worked with Robert Koch in Berlin but split with him over Koch's insistence that the only form real tuberculosis could take was its bacillary form. Babes, who also worked with Pasteur, knew better. Moreover, Babèş was fully aware of the void that Koch, the discoverer of tuberculosis, had purposely left for future scientists such as Oskar Fischer in validating forms such as the filamentous *Streptothrix*-like tuberculosis.

Yet subsequently, bacteriologists Vera and Rettger[19] of Yale openly contradicted Koch. Vera wrote, "The single point on which all investigators have agreed is that the Koch [tubercular] bacillus does not always manifest itself in the classical rod shape. While at times and most commonly the organism appears as a granular rod, coccoid bodies, filaments, and clubs are not rare."[21]

And just ten years before Oskar Fischer found Actinomycosis-like forms in Alzheimer's cerebral plaque, Babèş and immunologist Levaditi reported in *"On the Actinomycotic Shape of the Tuberculous Bacilli"* that typical Actinomyces-like clusters [Drüsen] with clubs appeared in the tissue of rabbits inoculated with tubercle bacilli beneath the dura mater of their brains.[20] Once introduced into the brain this way, reported Babes, TB bacilli not only branched out like the Actinomycosis such as *Streptothrix*, but they developed rosettes that were identical to the "drüsen" that Oskar Fischer spotted in Alzheimer's plaque.

NOTES

1. A. Alzheimer, H. Forstl, and R. Levy, an English translation of Alzheimer's 1911 paper "Uber Eigenartige Krankheitsfalle des Spateren Alters" ("On Certain Peculiar Diseases of Old Age"), *History of Psychiatry* 2 (1991): 71–101.

2. T. Simchowitz, "La Maldie d'Alzheimer et Son Rapport Avec la Demence Senile," *Encephale* 9 (1914): 218–31.

3. W. Spielmeyer, "Alzheimer's Lebenswenk," *Zeitschrift fur die Gesamte Neurologie und Psychiatrie* 22 (1916): 1–44.

4. J. F. Ballenger, *Self, Senility, and Alzheimer's Disease in Modern America* (Baltimore: Johns Hopkins University Press, 2006).

5. R. Katzman, "The Prevalence and Malignancy of Alzheimer Disease," *Archives of Neurology* 33 (1976): 217–8.

6. N. Dunn, M. Mullee, V. H. Perry, and C. Holmes, "Association between Dementia and Infectious Disease: Evidence from a Case-Control Study," *Alzheimer Disease & Associated Disorders* 19, no. 2 (April–June 2005): 91–4.

7. I. E. Nee and C. F. Lipppa, "Alzheimer's Disease in Twenty-Two Twin Pairs—Thirteen-Year Follow-Up: Hormonal, Infectious, and Traumatic Factors," *Dementia and Geriatric Cognitive Disorders* 10 (1999): 148–51.

8. C. J. Alteri, J. Xicahténcati-Cortes, S. Hess, G. Caballero-Olin, J. A. Giron, and R. L. Friedman, "Mycobacterium Tuberculosis Produces Pili during Human Infection," *Procedures of the National Academy of Sciences* 104, no. 12 (2007): 5145–50.

9. C. Tukel, R. P. Wilson, J. H. Nishimori, M, Pezeshki, B. A. Chromy, and A. J. Baumler, "Responses to Amyloids of Microbial and Host Origin Are Mediated through Toll-Like

Receptor 2 Cell Host and Microbe,"*Cell Host Microbe*.6 (July 23, 2009): 45–53.

10. M. Kidd, "Paired Helical Filaments in Electron Microscopy of Alzheimer's Disease," *Nature* 197 (1963): 192–3.

11. O. Fischer, "Miliare Nekrosen Mit Drusigen Wucherungen der Neurofibrillen, eine Regelmassige Veranderung der Hirnrinde bei Seniler Demenz," *Monatsschr f Psychiat Neurol* 22 (1907): 372; O. Fischer, "Miliary Necrosis with Nodular Proliferation of the Neurofibrils: A Common Change of the Cerebral Cortex in Senile Dementia," *Monatsschrift fur Psychiatrie und Neurologie*, vol. XXII, Th. Ziehen (ed). (Berlin: Karger, 1907), 361–72; In T*he Early Story of Alzheimer's Disease*, edited by Katherine Bick, Luigi Amaducci, and Giancarlo Pepeu (Padova: Liviana Press, 1987), 5–18.

12. M. Goedert, "Oskar Fischer and the Study of Dementia," *Brain* 132, no. 4 (April 2009): 1102–11.

13. C. J. Alteri, J. Xicahtencati-Cortes, S. Hess, G. Caballero-Olin, J. A. Giron, and R. L. Friedman," Mycobacterium Tuberculosis Produces Pili during Human Infection," *Proceedings of the National Academy of Sciences* 104, no. 12 (March 2007): 5145–50.

14. J. M. Leonard and R. M. des Prez, "Tuberculous Meningitis," *Infectious Disease Clinics of North America* 4, no. 4 (December 1990): 769–87.

15. P. Blocq and G. Marinescu G, "Sur les Lesions et la Pathogenie de L'epilepsie Dite Essentielle," *Sem. Med* 12 (1892): 445–6.

16. G. Marinesco, *Anatomical and Clinical Study of the So-Called Senile Plaques*, 1er semestre, (Paris: Encephale, 1912), 105–32.

17. A. Chantemesse, "Étude Sur la Méningite Tuberculeuse de L'adulte: Les Formes Anormales en Particulier These de Medecine de Paris," no. 124 (1884).

18. P. Blocq, V. Babes, and G. Marinesco, *Atlas der Pathologischen Histologie des Nervensystems* (Berlin: Hirschwald, 1892).

19. H. D. Vera and L. F. Rettger, "Morphological Variation of the Tubercle Bacillus and Certain Recently Isolated Soil Acid Fasts, with Emphasis on Filterability," *Journal of Bacteriology* 39, no. 6 (June 1940): 659–87.

20. V. Babes and C. et Levaditi, "On the Actinomycotic Shape of the Tuberculosis Bacilli" ("Sur la Forme Actinomycosique du Bacilli de la Tuberculosis"), In *Arch. of Med. Exp. et D'anat*, part 2, 9, no. 6 (1897): 1041–8.

CHAPTER 2

Neurology Clinic, Salpêtrière Hospital, Paris, France, 1892

After Gheorghe Marinescu had worked for eminent bacteriologist Victor Babèş for several years, Babes arranged a valuable government scholarship that enabled Marinescu to study under Jean-Martin Charcot in Paris. There, Marinescu met Paul Blocq.

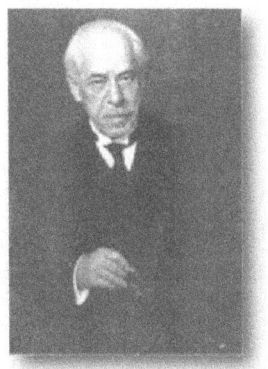 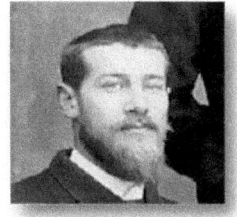

Figure 10. Gheorghe Marinescu.   Figure 11. Paul Oscar Blocq.

By 1892, Blocq and Marinescu described, for the first time, senile plaques as microglial nodules (see fig. 12) in the cerebral gray matter of nine deceased epileptic patients with histories of seizures.[1] Blocq and Marinescu did not relate such plaque to dementia, as Oskar Fischer did. Nor did Blocq and Marinescu stipulate what specifically might have caused such plaque, other than possibly brain microglia.

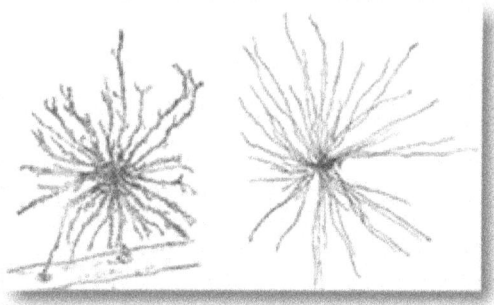

Figure 12. Microglia, or "glia," of the brain, which attack infection.
But once "activated" by such infection, common parlance claims that
such microglia can produce factors that are "detrimental" to neurons.
To Blocq and Marinescu, the source of Alzheimer's plaque was surrounding small cells comprised of microglia. But the possibility of an
underlying infection attacking and therefore altering such microglia
was something that Blocq and Marinescu, as well as many subsequent
investigators, ignored.

Nevertheless, Blocq and Marinescu were first to describe, upon
histological examination of epileptic brains, such "small nodules" that were later named "senile plaque." Marinescu described
what he found:

> Scattered throughout the various layers of the [brain's]
> cortex, small round clusters with a diameter of about
> 60μm, distinguished from the rest of the tissue by a much
> more intense staining, and regular contours. They thus
> appear as vaguely dotted structures sprinkling the back-
> ground of the slices. This is why it is possible to consider
> some of them at least as true multiple glial nodules. (?)[1]

Historians largely ignored the fact that this was just a hypotheti-
cal question within a statement, and they went on to imply that,

without reservation, Blocq and Marinescu thought such plaque nodules were of microglial origin alone. But even if that were the case, what underpinning factor, process, or infection(s) caused microglia to create such nodules?

Microglia are valuable elements in the brain's immune system. The fact is that the central nervous system (CNS) can be invaded and damaged by a variety of microorganisms. Indeed, the body's defense against such infections involves resident cells of the CNS, particularly microglia. However, it is only when microglia are activated by infection or inflammation that they produce "factors" that are detrimental and destructive to brain neurons[2] in a culture, creating, among other things, cerebral plaque. Microglia therefore are not in themselves the underlying cause of Alzheimer's plaque. More probably, an infection capable of entering them intracellularly and altering their architecture and metabolism is.

A distinctive characteristic of infection with *M. tuberculosis*, a disease that according to WHO (the World Health Organization) affects a third of the world, is its capacity to enter and replicate within macrophages in the blood. Within the brain, microglial cells are the resident macrophages. As such, human microglial cells are productively infected with *M. tuberculosis* and are, in fact, its principal target in the CNS.[3–5]

And just as the microglia are TB's principal target in the brain, microglia themselves are central to the response to the brain's response to fight cerebral TB.[6] Once infected, microglia can then serve as a reservoir of tuberculosis, surviving and possibly creating a pool or source of infection for further tubercular

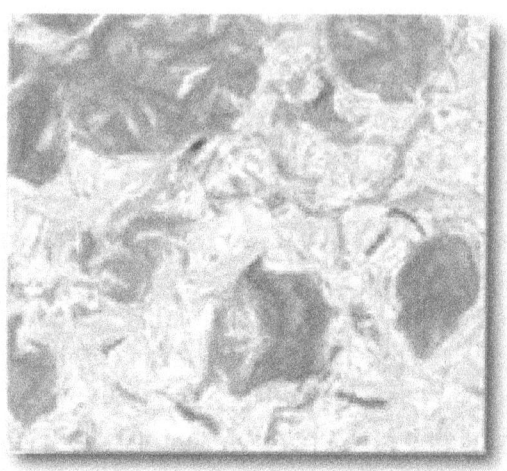

Figure 13. Circling in for the kill. Numerous tuberculous bacilli—relatively straight, rod-shaped bacilli (see arrow)—invading the cytoplasm of microglial (glial) cells from the base of the brain (1000 x magnification).

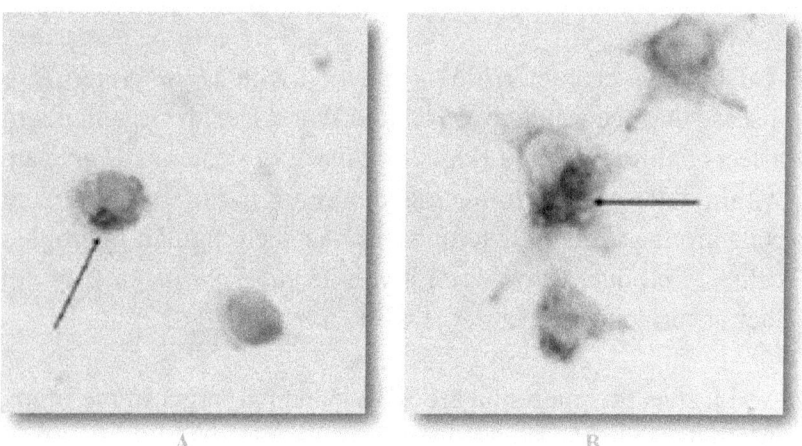

Figure 14. TB infecting microglia. (A) Taken after thirty minutes of tubercular Infection, followed by (B) at eighteen hours, which shows the retraction of microglial processes (1000x magnification).

attack in the brain.[3] For all of these reasons, microglia have emerged as being key to understanding the neuropathogenesis of tuberculosis in the CNS. When TB attacks and infects the microglia in the brain, unlike most pathogens, it at first resides quite comfortably in the microglia's cytoplasm within round, fluid-filled vacuoles, surviving and multiplying. Thus, TB and fowl-TB (avian tuberculosis) create their own cerebral infectious reservoirs. A short time later in such tubercular infection of the microglia, there is a retraction of the microglial processes. Tuberculosis will now direct a frontal offensive toward the brain's immune system, its virulent strains looking to inhibit the very defensive microglial cytokines that are so deadly to most other microbes.[7]

By 1910, Fischer, using staining techniques more advanced than either Redlich's or Blocq and Marinescu's, was able to demonstrate that senile plaques were not proliferating glial cells but rather a particular type of deposit of independent nature that subsequently "has been shown to have an outer area of degenerated neurons, a middle zone of swollen axons and dendrites, and a central amyloid core."[8]

The fact that Blocq and Marinescu never really probed a bacterial cause underlying their senile plaque in aged epileptics was characteristic of the way they did things. Thus, even in their watershed Parkinson's disease study, which formed much of our present concept of that disease, and after having established an attack by tuberculosis on the victim's *substantia nigra* (a brain structure located in the mesencephalon, or midbrain, that plays an important role in reward, addiction, and movement) they concluded that it was *substantia* pathology itself, not tuberculosis, that was behind their patient contracting Parkinson's.[9] The pathology of Parkinson's, other than its preference for the *substantia nigra*, is not unlike that of Alzheimer's. Neurologists Joynt and Griggs said this:

> Patients with idiopathic [of unknown origin] Parkinson's disease may also have diffuse cortical atrophy [as found in Alzheimer's]. In a study of this problem, it was found that all patients with Parkinson's disease had more cortical degeneration and more dementia than patients of similar age without Parkinson's disease. This observation suggests that Parkinson's disease is a diffuse, degenerative brain disease. When dementia is marked, the changes in the brain outside the *substantia nigra* may be similar to those found in Alzheimer's disease, including senile plaques and neurofibrillary tangles, suggesting that dementia in some forms of parkinsonism may be variants [modifications] of senile dementia of the Alzheimer type.[10]

Blocq and Marinescu's historical Parkinson's patient was a thirty-eight-year-old male with a tubercular mass (tuberculoma) the size and shape of a filbert nut, lodged in his right midbrain. This mass had destroyed the two small, linear configurations at the bottom of his brain, the *substantia nigra*. Once these were damaged, this right-sided midbrain mass effectively left him with left-sided Parkinson's from the crossover that nerves take on their way from the brain to the spine.

The fact that this man died from pulmonary tuberculosis was never a question in either Blocq or Marinescu's mind. Before uncovering the tubercular brain mass, Blocq opened the deceased's chest and saw that the vertebral portions of his first and second ribs were completely eaten away as a result of spread from a tubercular lung.

Blocq and Marinescu persisted in their anti-infectious theory, despite their knowledge that their mentor, Charcot, had documented a second case of Parkinson's from TB, just as Mendel had in his paper[11] about a child with parkinsonian tremors who died of tuberculosis. Blocq had also read Krafft Ebing's study, in which a tubercular mass in the midbrain also led to Parkinson's. Levy–Valensi[12] then published a case on the extreme rigidity and a Parkinsonian stare in a young woman with cerebral TB. And soon thereafter, Scheinker[13] from Vienna weighed in with his own case of Parkinson's as a result of the tubercular encephalitis inflaming his patient's brain. Not only did Wilder[14] observe Parkinson's in the course of severe lung tuberculosis, but his autopsy showed that the diffuse degeneration of the brain's parenchyma simulated Alzheimer's, except for its peculiar preference for the *substantia nigra*. Yet in his description of the extent of the tubercular infection affecting his patient's brain, Wilder mentioned that any tubercular gross lesions spotted were completely outside the CNS. This brought up the possibility of immunological-based neuronal damage from a focus of the disease outside of the brain. Almost in answer to Blocq and Marinescu's microglial quest, Simmonds[13] of England, among others, showed that the brain's microglia could be attacked by tuberculosis until their central parts were destroyed, leaving plaque and other pathology as a result. Hadn't Sittig[15] pointed out that even the smallest neuroglia (glia) and ganglions of the brain showed a falling apart under tubercular attack? Alzheimer himself knew that CNS diseases such as Parkinson's and Alzheimer's could be the same disease process simply affecting different parts of the brain. Alzheimer said this:

> An identical disease process will be able to cause extraordinarily different clinical features because of differences in its localization, and in the sequence and extent of cortical involvement, which may be diffuse or localized and moreover possible localized in many different ways.[16]

Blocq and Marinesco might never have connected the dots regarding why microglia might spawn senile plaque beyond their changed microglial architecture. But Marinesco's[17] haunting drawing, detailing the anatomical study of senile plaque, uncannily resembles the microbial attack (with drüsen) laid out for Alzheimer's by Oskar Fischer.

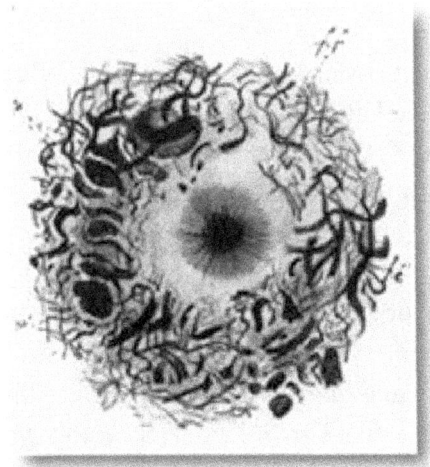

Figure 15. One of Marinescu's drawings from his Anatomical and Clinical Study of the So-Called Senile Plaques, Marinescu G. (1912), Encephale (Paris), 1er semestre, pp. 105–32. This drawing depicts senile plaque using silver stain with an outer layer of fibers that are short and thick with other thinner fibers present. Some are almost club-shaped, as in the drüsen of Oskar Fischer.

NOTES

1. P. Blocq and G. Marinescu, "Sur les Lesions et la Pathogenie de L'epilepsie Dite Essentielle," *Sem Med* 12 (1892): 445–6.

2. D. Giulian, K. Vaca, and M. Corpuz, "Brain Glia Release Factors with Opposing Actions upon Neuronal Survival," *Journal of Neuroscience* 13 (1993): 29–37.

3. M. Curto, C. Reali, G. Palmieri, F. Scintu, Schivo, et al., "Inhibition of Cytokines Expression in Human Microglia Infected with Virulent and Nonvirulent Mycobacteria," *Neurochemistry International* 44 (2004): 381–92.

4. R. B. Rock, G. Gekker, S. Hu, W. S. Sheng, M. Cheeran, et al, "Role of Microglia in Central Nervous System Infections," *Clinical Microbial Reviews* 17 (2004): 942–64.

5. P. K. Peterson, G. Gekker, S. Hu, W. S. Sheng, et al., "CD14 Receptor-Mediated Uptake of Nonopsonized Mycobacterium Tuberculosis by Human Microglia," *Infection and Immunity* 63, no. 4 (April 1995): 1598–602.

6. J. A. Green, P. T. Elkington, C. J. Pennington, F. Roncaroli, S. Dholakia, et al., "Mycobacterium Tuberculosis Upregulates Microglial Matrix Metalloproteinase-1 and -3 Expression and Secretion via NF-kappaB- and Activator Protein-1-Dependent Monocyte Networks," *Journal of Immunology* 184, no. 11 (June 1, 2010): 6492–503.

7. E. Beltan, L. Horgen, and N. Rastogi, "Secretion of Cytokines by Human Macrophages upon Infection by Pathogenic and Nonpathogenic Mycobacteria, *Microbiology and Pathology* 28 (2000): 313–8.

8. O. Fischer, "Die Presbyophrene Demenz, Deren Anatomische Grundlage und Klinische Abgrenzung," *Z. Ges. Neurol. Psychiat.* 3 (1910): 371–471.

9. P. Blocq and G. Marinesco, "Sur un Cas de Tremblement Parkinsonien he'Miple'Gique Symptomatique d'une Tumeur du Pe'Doncule ce'Re' Bral," *Mem. Soc. Biol.* 5 (1893): 105–11.

10. Joynt RJ, Griggs RC. The Extrapyramidal System and Disorders of Movement. In *Clinical Neurology* Revised Edition 1996. Lippincott-Raven Publishers. Philadelphia New York. Vol 3: 38:23-24.

11. "Mendel: Berliner Klinische Wochensrift," no. 29. 1885,

12. J. Levy-Valensi, "Meningite Tuberculeuse Ayam un Syndrome Parkinsonien," *Semaine des Hopitaux de Paris*, no. 20 (December 31, 1931): 653–4.

13. I. Scheinker, *Encephalitis Tuberculosa im Striatom-unter dem Bilde eines Parkinsonismus. Deutsche Zeitschrift fur Nervenheil Kunde.* (Berlin: Veriage Bon FCW Vogel, 1936).

14. J. Wilder, *Mschr. Psychiatv 61* (1926).

15. O. Sittig, Befunde mit Hertwig-Magendiescher Augeneinstellung *Neurology* Vol. 2–3 (1914).

16. A. Alzheimer, H. Forstl, and R. Levy, an English translation of Alzheimer's 1911 paper "Uber Eigenartige Krankheitsfalle des Spateren Alters" ("On Certain Peculiar Diseases of Old Age"), *History of Psychiatry* 2 (1991): 93.

17. G. Marinesco, "Etude Anatomique et Clinique des Plaques Dites Seniles, 1er semestre Encephale (Paris), 1912, 105–132.

CHAPTER 3

Office of the Editor, Monatsschrift fuer Psychiatrie und Neurologie at S. Karger, Berlin, 1907

First accepted and published in 1907, Fischer's twelve-case Alzheimer's paper[1] was far superior to Alois Alzheimer's short, single-case nondiagrammatic paper reporting both tangles and plaques. Alzheimer's 1907 paper was a brief transcript of a short speech he gave in Tubingen in December of the previous year. In contrast, Fischer's paper was a detailed description of senile plaque, offering as a control to his cases with senile dementia the analysis of the brains of ten normal individuals, ten with psychosis only, and forty-five more with neurosyphilis of the brain. But of all of these, only in the specimens with age-related dementia did Fischer find senile plaque. He did not find senile plaque in neurosyphilis.

Faced with a disease that then, very much as now, yielded a shrunken brain dotted with amyloid plaque among its neurons, Fischer found Alzheimer's "tangles" only 21 percent of the time. He concluded that it was plaque, not tangles, that were responsible for the age-related dementias. He tirelessly autopsied hundreds of cases to prove this.

Yet to be certain, it was Fischer's regard for Alzheimer's plaque as the expression of a possible specific infectious cause that put him in a place that few others, including Alzheimer, dared to go.

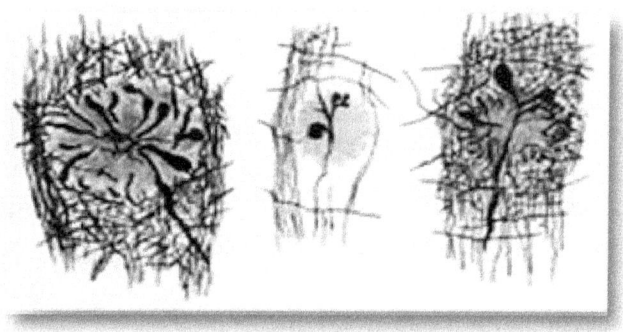

Figure 16. Fischer's more detailed drawings of Alzheimer brain plaque. Once again, abnormal, club-shaped neurons grow and displace normal-looking fibrils in the space occupied by the plaques. In evidence again are the club-shaped, black "drüsen" that can result from infection with either TB or actinomycosis (Aktinomycesdruse).

The tenth edition of Ziegler's classical German text, *Pathology*,[2] which Fischer used as a reference, mentions that the actino-mycosis like *Streptothrix* and tuberculosis were so similar that Lubarsch and others insisted that the two be classified together.[3] Lubarsch contended this only after first confirming Victor Babes's study. Choppen-Jones went so far as to propose that tuberculosis be called "tuberculomycosis."[4] And Zeigler's mention of Babes's study forced its entry into a 1910 edition of *Lippincott's*, which cautioned that tubercle bacilli occurred "as small branching complexes resembling the "drüsen" of the actinomyces."[5]

So it becomes all but obvious that Fischer's 1907 por-trayal of Alzheimer plaque as often appearing like bacterial "Streptotriches" had to be weighed within the context that *Streptothrix* was linked to, confused with, and often indistin-guishable from tuberculosis. Therefore, when Fischer found that nearly all brain plaque in the 60 to 80μ microscopic range had an appearance reminiscent of "glandular" actinomyces, American bacteriologist Davis mentioned that Fischer's "glandular" actinomycosis were among the most difficult to differentiate from tuberculosis: "the two are often all but indistinguishable."[6]

By 1907, Oskar Fischer even went to the extent of saying that many of the senile plaques he found "resemble more closely the central cell-free part of a tubercle."[1] A tubercle, or the tuberculoma it eventually forms, is a small nodule that very often forms in brain tissue after the bloodborne spread of miliary tuberculosis. The very title of Fischer's paper mentions a tubercular-like "miliary necrosis" of nerve fibrils in the brain in the age-related dementias.

In his papers, Oskar Fischer refers to the minute nodules and granules inside diseased, mature Alzheimer's plaque as either "drüsen," "drusige nekrosen" (necrotic drüsen), or simply "miliare nekrosen" (miliary necrosis). The latter term would eventually come to represent cerebral amyloid.[7] In his *Pathology* textbook at that time, Zeigler talked at length of amyloid, seeing it as usually a complication of chronic tuberculosis or perhaps syphilis.[2]

It has been known for almost a century that chronic bacterial infections, prominently tuberculosis, could be associated with amyloid deposition.[8] In other words, there was a time when it was considered that to have amyloidosis or beta-amyloidosis was to have tuberculosis. It took Divry three decades of knockdown, drag-out struggles before the medical establishment of his day would acknowledge amyloid's role in the neurodegenerative diseases, including Alzheimer's. And later, neuropathologist Philip Schwartz of Warren, Pennsylvania, who helped Divry prevail, concluded that despite the invention of "newer" amyloid classification systems, tuberculosis could still safely be considered the most frequent infection that induces the formation of amyloid in human pathology.[9]

There can no longer be any serious doubt that the Congo-red-dye-stained, beta-pleated sheets found in Alzheimer's amyloid fibrils can be generated by amyloid producing bacteria-like tuberculosis.[10] And it has been established that the production of amyloid is all over the footprint of the mycobacteria, including *Mycobacterium tuberculosis*, a disease that Alteri and others estimate to be responsible for nearly three million human deaths worldwide.[11] Despite the WHO's conservative estimates, Fox[12] maintained that "Nearly half the world's population is infected with TB."

Recently, Alteri showed[11] that during active infection, *M. tuberculosis* produces outer fringelike bacterial amyloid structures called "fimbriae" or "pilli" on its surface that also bind Congo red dye, a property associated with human amyloidosis. Such beta-amyloid TB manufactured pilli have crucial roles in infection, one of which is to allow tuberculosis to adhere to or stick onto targeted immune cells, including the microglia (neuroglia) in the nervous system. Once colonized, such microglia can in turn can act as their own reservoir to spread infection.

Moreover, Jordal[13] reconfirmed that mycobacteria like TB produce a level of amyloid not previously described for any other bacteria. Not only was amyloid found present in mycobacterial biofilms, but in the actual cell envelops of the mycobacteria, as well as coating the spores they produce.

By 1984, de Beer[14], studying the relationship between a major rise of serum amyloid and having tuberculosis, also saw a rapid descent in amyloid in patients treated with antitubercular drugs. As an offshoot of de Beer's work, Tomiyama[15] dissolved ß-amyloid plaque with rifampin, a first-line drug in the treatment of TB, and one of the few agents, to this day, that is able to dissolve amyloid plaque.

While Oskar Fischer pondered his findings in Prague, Edith Claypole, in far-off Berkley, California, wrote that the "drüsen" of Fischer and earlier German writers, with their characteristic, frequent club-shaped forms, were simply small, separate colonies of either tuberculosis or closely related actinomyces. Claypole wrote the following analysis:

> The "drüsen" and their clubs are now recognized as being the result of a reaction between the microorganism [TB or an actinomycosis-like *Streptothrix*] and the tissues of the host, rather than essential morphologic features.[16]

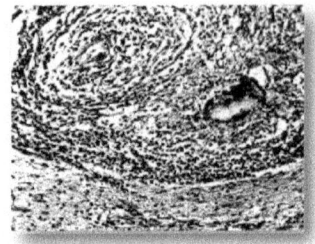

Figure 17. Appearance of the brain's frontal cortex with tubercular meningeal tissue. The exudate is chiefly of round cells—cells similar to what many of the early Alzheimer's investigators were seeing.

In the same year that Oskar Fischer finished his final ground-breaking paper on Alzheimer-like dementia, US investigator Hubert Williams isolated both TB and *actinomycosis* (*Streptothrix*) from a case of tubercular pericarditis, reporting it in what was subsequently called *The American Journal of Pathology*. Williams wrote, "Even in the face of the evidence stated, the writer still finds himself questioning whether or not the tubercle bacillus may not yet become a typical *Streptothrix* under certain conditions now unknown."[17]

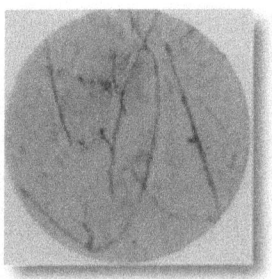

Figure 18. Williams's slide of tubercle bacilli, grown on 1 percent dextrose serum, in the incubator for one week, with round spore forms just beginning to develop. Note that Williams's description of "long, tangled threads" is similar to that for Streptothrix [actinomycosis] below.

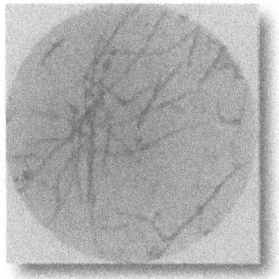

Figure 19. Williams's slide of actinomycosis [Streptothrix] in its sporulating phase with accompanying round spores. Such filamentous forms are extremely similar to those seen in the tubercular filamentous forms of fig. 18.

So Hubert Williams joined the chorus of other investigators who saw TB and *Streptothrix* assume identical forms.

NOTES

1. O. Fischer, "Miliary Necrosis with Nodular Proliferation of the Neurofibrils, a Common Change of the Cerebral Cortex in Senile Dementia," *Monatsschrift fuer Psychiatrie und Neurologie*, vol. XXII, edited by Th. Ziehen (Berlin: S. Karger, 1907), 361–72.

2. E. Zeigler, "General Pathology Translated from the Tenth Revised German Edition, edited by Alfred Scott Warthin, MD, (New York: William Wood and Company, 1903), 757.

3. D. Lubarsch, "Zur Kenntn: D. Strahlenpilze," xxxi, *Zeitschr. f. Hyg.*, (1899).

4. A. Coppen-Jones, "Uber die Nomanklature des Sogenannten: Tuberkalbacillus," in *Centralbl. f. Bacteriol. l, Abt., v.*20, no. 10/11 (1896): 393–5.

5. H. W. Cattell, *Lippincott's New Medical Dictionary* (Philadelphia and London: J. B. Lippincott Company, 1910): 1033, 1108.

6. D. J. Davis, "Some Observations on *Streptothrix* Infections and Their Relation to Tuberculosis in the National Association for the Study and Prevention of Tuberculosis," *Transactions of the Eleventh Annual Meeting, Seattle, Washington, June 14–16, 1915* (Baltimore: Williams & Wilkins Company, 1935), 255–61.

7. W. Scholz, "Studien zur Pathologie der Hirngefa sse II: Die drusige Entartung der Hirnarterien und—Capillaren," *Z. ges. Neurol. Psychiat.*(1938) 162, 694–715.

8. Z. S. Khachaturian, "Diagnosis of Alzheimer's Disease," *Archives of Neurology & Psychiatry* 42 (1985): 1097–1105.

9. P. Schwartz, "Amyloid Degeneration and Tuberculosis in the Aged," *Gerontologia* 18, no. 5–6 (1972): 321–62.

10. L. Wang, S. K. Maji, M. R. Sawaya, M. R. Eisenberg, and R. Riek, "Bacterial Inclusion Bodies Contain Amyloid-Like Structure," *PLOS Biology* 6, no. 8 (August 5, 2008): e195.

11. C. J. Alteri, J. Xicahténcati-Cortes, S. Hess, G. Caballero-Olin, J. A. Girón, and R. L. Friedman, "Mycobacterium Tuberculosis Produces Pili during Human Infection," *Proceedings of the National Academy of Sciences* 104, no. 12 (March 20, 2007): 5145–50.

12. J. L. Fox, "TB: A Grim Disease of Numbers," *ASM News* 56 (1990): 363–4.

13. P. B. Jordal, et al., "Widespread Abundance of Functional Bacterial Amyloid in Mycolata and Other Gram-Positive Bacteria," *Applied and Environmental Microbiology* (June 2009), p. 4101-4110.

14. F. C. De Beer and A. E. Nel, "Serum Amyloid A-Protein and C - reactive protein Levels in Pulmonary Tuberculosis: Relationship to Amyloidosis," *Thorax* 30, no. 3 (1984):196–200.

15. T. Tomiyama, A. Satoshi, "Rifampicin Prevents the Aggregation and Neurotoxicity of Amyloid B Protein *in vitro*," *Biochemical and Biophysical Research Communications* 2014, no. 1 (1994): 76–83.

16. E. J. Claypole, "*Streptothrix* Infections and Their Differentiation from Tuberculosis," in *The National Association for the Study and Prevention of Tuberculosis: Transactions of the Tenth Annual Meeting, Washington, DC, May 7–8, 1914* (Philadelphia: Wm. F. Fell Company, 1914): 169.

17. H. U. Williams, "A Pleomorphic Bacillus Growing in Association with a *Streptothrix*," *Journal of Medical Research* 27:2 (1912): 157–161.

CHAPTER 4

Nervenklinik, Department of Clinical Psychiatry, University of Munich, Munich, Germany, 1907

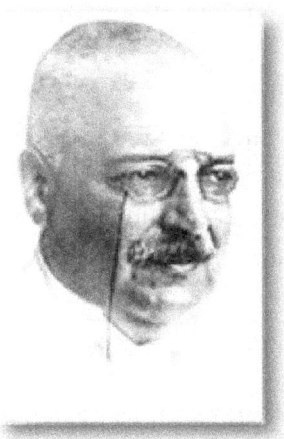

Figure 20. In search of a post where he could combine research and clinical practice, Alois Alzheimer (1864–1915) became research assistant to Emil Kraepelin at the Munich medical school in 1903. There he created a new laboratory for brain research.

In the form of Oskar Fischer, Alois Alzheimer and Emil Kraepelin soon realized that they had a huge problem. Alzheimer acknowledged the importance of Fischer's plaques in Alzheimer's disease. Nevertheless, Alzheimer had to try to make his case that his findings were somehow different from Fischer's. And to do so unfortunately would, in part, require raising some doubt regarding Fischer's thoughts and findings. Thus, by 1911 Alzheimer wrote the following:

> Hitherto opinions about the nature of the plaques have been very divergent. Fischer pointed out their similarity to bacterial colonies and reported that he had undertaken cultivation experiments and complement-fixation tests which however produced negative results.[1]

At the time Fischer undertook cultivation and compliment fixation tests to validate his germ, negative results were the rule, not the exception. Alzheimer should have known this. Thus, the fact that Fischer's cultivation experiments and complement fixations were negative did not rule out the existence of Fischer's brain microbe.

For example, in the same year that Alzheimer made his 1911 statement, Harbitz and Grondahl reported repeatedly negative attempts at running complement-fixation tests in all cases using the serum of patients with known *Streptothrix* (actinomycosis) patients.[2] Before that, Woodhead, Director of Laboratories at the Royal College of Physicians, pointed out that any attempted failure to cultivate *Streptothrix* could easily occur when trying to cultivate the well-developed club-shaped form of the organism that Fischer repeatedly documented. Woodhead wrote this about such experiments:

> It is interesting to note that most of the experiments that have been made on the cultivation of this organism [*Streptothrix*] have been attended with complete

failure—a failure that in some measure, at any rate, appears to be due to the fact that almost all experimenters have used for their inoculating material only those colonies in which the club-shaped [*Streptothrix*] organisms have become well developed. The first attempt that was at all successful was made by Bostrom, who, throwing aside the club-like processes, took for his inoculating material the central network, selecting as far as possible young growing colonies for his seed material."[3]

But even Bostrom succeeded in getting only eleven positive growths out of several hundred planted.[4]

And when German investigator Fritzsche[5] addressed this same topic three years before Alzheimer challenged Fischer's microorganism, Fritzsche found not only a limited number of cases in which complement fixation for *Streptothrix* proved positive, but, in addition, there were frequent cross-reactions in his meager positive test samples for *Streptothrix* with tuberculosis. He added that *Streptothrix* was further confused with TB because they both could stain with tubercular acid-fast dyes, and both could have filamentous as well as club-like forms. But Bolton[6] later pointed out that unlike TB, Fischer's *Streptothrix* rarely involved the central nervous system. Furthermore, although the first case of *Streptothrix* involving the CNS was reported by Ponfick[7] in 1882, Harz never succeeded in cultivating the organism from there.[8] Most of this literature was readily available to the Alzheimer group.

Moreover, even in the case of using complement-fixation tests to detect the far, far more prevalent tuberculosis, Corper[9] reported as late as 1916 that such tests were positive in only 30 percent of already-proven cases of tuberculosis—whether active or inactive.

Although Oskar Fischer's name was associated with the discovery of the mechanism of memory loss in senile dementia (presbyophrenia), as we now know, he was also the co-discoverer of "Alzheimer's disease." And there is more than enough evidence that Alzheimer himself knew that there was no fundamental difference between his "presenile dementia" and Fischer's "senile" (over the age of sixty-five) dementia. At one point, even Alzheimer spark-plug Perusini admitted that "these morbid forms do not represent anything but atypical form of senile dementia."[10] But senile dementia, atypical or not, already had a name: Fischer's disease.

Yet Alzheimer's superior, Emil Kraepelin, one of the most politically powerful psychiatrists of all time, would not hear it. Soon Kraepelin would classify Alzheimer's "presenile" dementia on page 627 in the eighth edition of his influential *Textbook of Psychiatry* (1910)[11], without any reference to the fact that similar findings by Fischer had appeared previous to the Alzheimer study.[12]

Despite being the painstaking, technically and descriptively flawless neuropathologist Alzheimer was, the exact nature of the cause for the disease named after him remained totally elusive to him. And his 1907 paper on Alzheimer's was remarkable not because it advanced the knowledge or reason behind cerebral plaque or because it pointed to a possible specific cause as Fischer's microbial hypothesis had, but rather because it described—in addition to Fischer's plaque—Alzheimer's tangles and other pathological points of interest in the affected brain.

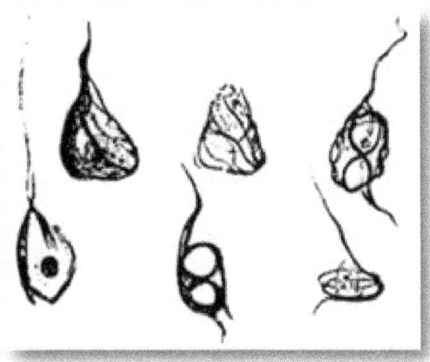

Figure 21. Tangles in the neurofibrils of the brain, drawn by Alzheimer. From ref. 9 in the eighth edition of Kraepelin's Handbook of Psychiatry (E. Kraepelin, Psychiatrie, eighth ed. Vol I: Allgemeine Psychiatrie; Vol II: Klinische Psychiatrie (Barth: Leipzig, Germany, 1909–10.)

However, others had spotted and documented such tangles (neurofibrillary degeneration) earlier than Alzheimer, including Fragnito[13] in 1904, Bianchi[14] in 1906, and Fuller in 1907.[15]

Meanwhile, nothing spoke more of the continued heavy hand of Alzheimer's chief Kraepelin than that long before Kraepelin formally codified Alzheimer's "presenile" dementia, it was Binswanger, in 1898, who had first introduced the term "presenile dementia." One year later, Kraepelin adopted the term for his own *Compendium der Psychiatrie*, where it remained until Kraepelin decided it was time to assign it the name "Alzheimer's disease."

Had it been Oskar Fischer alone who expressed his dismay at the absurdity of Kraepelin's distinction of "presenile" from "senile" dementia, that would have been notable. But similar objections were also raised by Fuller,[16] Hakkebousch in Russia,[17] Lugaro,[18] and Lambert[19]—all of whom questioned Alzheimer's as a separate disease. Alzheimer was all too familiar with the objections. Alzheimer noted the following:

> The question arises whether these cases of disease, which I have considered peculiar, still show characteristic features in clinical and histological aspects that distinguish them from senile dementia or whether they must be assigned instead to senile dementia itself.[1]

Be that as it may, on November 3, 1906, Alois Alzheimer traveled to the auditorium of the Clinic for Psychiatry at the University of Tubingen, Germany, to present and describe the pathological characteristics of his "unusual" case of dementia. Alzheimer's deceased patient, Auguste Deter, would soon become known as the first documented case of Alzheimer's disease (AD)—but not right away. At this presentation, Alzheimer also described other aspects of Deter's autopsy, specifically the staining of abnormal neurons in her brain:

> Because these fibrils were stained differently from normal neurofibrils, a chemical conversion of the neurofibrils must have occurred. This may well explain why the fibrils survived the decay of cells."[20]

Yes, a chemical conversion. But from what? First there were technical considerations concerning the stain used. Key to

Alzheimer and Oskar Fischer being able to find Alzheimer's pathology was their use of the reduced silver staining technique developed by Max Bielschowsky.[21,22] Bielschowsky's stain impregnated silver into nerve fibers using chemicals shared by photographers, Bielschowsky believed he had come across a reliable way to stain what he was already referring to as "neurofibrils." Indeed, when both Alzheimer and Fischer used the stain, they noticed increased staining in many of the brain's pathological cortical nerve cells. Alzheimer's assistant, Gaetano Perusini, praised Bielschowsky's method, observing that "by this method the plaques are seen impregnated more or less intensely with silver nitrate."[23]

But silver stains are also known to be very sensitive in the staining of bacteria and apparently unknown to Bielschowsky, silver nitrate also binds to the outer layers of the tubercle bacilli, allowing its visualization as well. By 1911, Von Getegh had described a method showing that silver nitrate brought tubercular spores into sharp relief. Early on, Egons Darzins,[24] who later worked at the Robert Koch Institute in Berlin, recognized that tubercular bacilli could be stained with silver nitrate.

Another clue to the "chemical conversion of the neurofibrils" that Alzheimer stipulated surfaced in 2004, approximately one hundred years after Alzheimer's presentation in Tubingen. German scientists, working mere blocks away from where Alzheimer gave his talk, established that the renegade protein called "tau"—constituting at least in part the chemical conversion that Alzheimer was trying to describe—could be generated in the brains of laboratory animals inoculated with tubercular elements.[25] If normal tau protein nourished a neuron's axon, the abnormal "hyperphosphorylated" tau after mycobacterial attack formed sticky clumps, much like what happened with Alzheimer's beta-amyloid plaque, resulting in the death of the neuron. Tuberculosis itself contains a phosphatide fraction with 3 percent phosphorus and has the ability to phosphorylate CNS tissues, including neurons.[26] Not only can TB produce the same protein phosphorylation[27,28] seen in autopsied Alzheimer's brains,[29] but the very same inflammatory neurotoxic proteinase and cytokines instrumental in the creation of beta-amyloid plaque, tau aggregation, and neurofibrillary tangles in Alzheimer's[30] are operative and found elevated also in the phosphorylated tissue specimens from patients with CNS tuberculosis.[26]

Just prior to Alzheimer and Fischer—in the second half of the nineteenth century—biomedicine had witnessed explosive growth, with Germany at its epicenter. Central to this was microscopy, the cellular doctrine of Rudolf Virchow, and its application in the bacteriology of Robert Koch, who discovered the TB bacillus. It was in this research setting that Alzheimer initiated his own probes, hardly mentioning Koch at a time when an estimated one-quarter of the adult population of Europe was dying from TB.[31] At the same time, Alzheimer was initially limited by the extreme dogma of Virchow, which stated that amyloid, a known by-product of Koch's tuberculosis, did not form in the central nervous system. How influential this erroneous doctrine was on generations of pathologists cannot be underestimated. Because of Virchow's severe miscalculation, Alzheimer's initial conception arose of a "cerebral colloidal degeneration" going on in Alzheimer's brains, hindering the recognition of the real nature of cerebral plaque and deposits.

As late as 1930, Lubarsch wrote the following:

> It is not emphasized enough that, as it seems, amyloid never affects the central nervous system; this fact has already come to the attention of Virchow. I, myself, in spite of particular circumspection, in cases of most intense generalized amyloidosis, have never found even traces of amyloid [in the brain].[32]

How wrong this would prove to be.

NOTES

1. A. Alzheimer, H. Forstl, and R. Levy, an English translation of Alzheimer's 1911 paper "Uber Eigenartige Krankheitsfalle des Spateren Alters" ("On Certain Peculiar Diseases of Old Age"), *History of Psychiatry* 2 (1991): 71–101.

2. F. Harbitz and N. B. Grondahl, "Actinomycosis in Norway: Studies in the Etiology, Modes of Infection, and Treatment," *American Journal of Medical Science* 142 (1911): 386–95.

3. G. S. Woodhead, *Bacteria and Their Products* (London and New York: Walter Scott, Ltd./Charles Scribner's Sons, 1895), 258

4. V. Z. Cope, "Actinomycosis: The Actinomyces and Some Common Errors about the actinomyces and actinomycosis." Postgraduate Medical Journal 28 (1952): 572–4

5. E. Fritzsche, "Experimentelle Untersuchungen Tiber Biologische Beziehungen des Tuberkelbazillus zu Einigen Anderen Saurefesten Mikroorganismen und Aktinomyzeten," *Archive for Hygiene* 5 (1908): 181–220.

6. C. F. Bolton and E. M. Ashenhurst, "Review Article: Actinomycosis of the Brain. *Canadian Medical Association Journal* 90 (April 11, 1964): 922–8.

7. E. Ponfick, Die Actinomykose des Menschen, Eine Neue Infectionskrankheit auf Vergleichend-Pathologischer und Experimenteller Grundlage Geschildert (Berlin: A. Hirschwald, 1882).

8. B. Harz, "Actinomyces Bovis, ein Neuer Schimmel in den Geweben des Rindes: Deutsche Zeitschr. f. their," *Med. und Vergl. Path.* (1870): 125, Zweites Supplementheft.

9. H. J. Corper, "Complement-Fixation in Tuberculosis," *The Journal of Infectious Diseases* 19, no. 3 (September 1916): 315–21.

10. G. Perusini, "Sul Valore Nosografico di Alcuni Reperti *Istopatologice Caratteristici per la Senilita,*" *Rivista Italiana di Neuropatologia* 4 (1911): 193–213.

11. E. Kraepelin, *Psychiatrie*, 8th ed., vol. I: *Allgemeine Psychiatrie*; vol. II: *Klinische Psychiatrie*(Leipzig, Germany: Barth, 1909–10).

12. M. Vojtechovsky, "The Roots of Old-Age Psychiatry in Prague," an abstract presented at the Fourteenth Conference of Alzheimer Europe in Prague, Prague, Czech Republic, May 20–23, 2004.

13. O. Fragnito, "Sur Quelques Alterations de L'appareil Neurofribillaire des Cellules Corticalesdans la Demence Senile," *Annals of Neurology* 22 (1904): 130–7.

14. L. Bianchi, *A Textbook of Psychiatry* (London: Balliere & Tyndall, 1906) and the American neuropathologist Fuller.

15. S. C. Fuller, "A Study of the Neurofibrils in Dementia Paralytica, Dementia Senilis, Chronic Alcoholism, Cerebral Lues, and Microcephalic Idiocy," American Journal of Insanity 63 (1907): 415–68.

16. S.C. Fuller, "Alzheimer's Disease (Seniumpraecox): The Report of a Case and Review of Published Cases," *Journal of Nervous and Mental Disease* 39 (1912):440–455, 536–557.

17. B. M. Hakkebousch and T. A. Geier, "De la Maladie d'Alzheimer," *Ann Med-Psychol* 71 (1913): 358.

18. E. Lugaro, "La Psichiatria Tedesca Nella Storia e Nell'Attualita," *Riv Patol Nerv Ment* 21 (1916–17): 241–283, 337–86, 449–501, 577–617; 22: 65–104, 185–239, 249–302.

19. Charles I. Lambert, "The Clinical and Anatomical Features of *Alzheimer's* Disease," *Journal of Nervous & Mental Disease* 44, no. 2 (August 1916): 169–70.

20. K. Maurer and U. Mauer, *Alzheimer 's disease: The Life of a Physician and the Career of a Disease* (Chichester, West Sussex: Columbia University Press, 2003).
21. M. Bielschowsky, "Die Silberimpragnation der Achsenzylinder," Centralbl 21 (1902): 578–84.
22. Bielschowsky M. Die Silberimpragnation der Neurofibrillen. *Centralbl* 1903; 22: 997–1006.
23. G. Perusini, "Uber Klinisch und Histologish Eigenartige Psychische Erkrankungen des Spateren Lebensalters," in Histologische und Histopathologische Arbeiten, edited by F. Nissl and A. Alzheimer (Jena, Germany: Verlag G. Fischer, 1909), 297–351.
24. E. Darzins, *The Bacteriology of Tuberculosis.* University of Minnesota Press (1958) 488 pp, 187.
25. A. Schneider, G. W. Arau'jo, K. Trajkovic, M. M. Herrmann, D. Merkler, E. Mandelkow, R. Weissert, and M. Simons, "Hyperphosphorylation and Aggregation of Tau in Experimental Autoimmune Encephalomyelitis," *The Journal of Biological Chemistry* 279, no. 53 (December 31, 2004): 55833–9.
26. J. E. Harris, M. Fernandez-Vilaseca, P. T. G. Elkington, D. E. Horncastle, M. B. Graeber, et al., "IFN Synergizes with IL-1to Up-Regulate MMP-9 Secretion in a Cellular Model of Central Nervous System Tuberculosis," *The FASEB Journal* 21 (February 2007): 356–65.
27. U. Kusebauch, C. Ortega, A. Ollodart, R. S. Rogers, D. R. Sherman, et al., "Mycobacterium Tuberculosis Supports Protein Tyrosine Phosphorylation," *Proceedings of the National Academy of Sciences* 111, no. 25 (June 24, 2014): 9265–70, doi: 10.1073/pnas.1323894111, e-pub 2014.

28. K. Chow, D. Ng, R. Stokes, and P. Johnson, "Protein Tyrosine Phosphorylation in Mycobacterium Tuberculosis," *FEMS Microbiology Letters* 124, no. 2 (December 1, 1994): 203–7.

29. I. P. Shapiro, E. Masliah, and T. Saitoh, "Altered Protein Tyrosine Phosphorylation in Alzheimer's Disease" *Journal of Neurochemistry* 56, no. 4 (April 1991): 1154–62.

30. X.-X. Wang, M.-S. Tan, J.-T. Yu, and L. Tan, "Matrix Metalloproteinases and Their Multiple Roles in Alzheimer's Disease," *BioMed Research International* 2014, article ID 908636, http://dx.doi.org/10.1155/2014/908636.

31. P. M. Simone and W. D. Samuel, "Multidrug-Resistant Tuberculosis," 1994 National Center for HIV/AIDS, Viral Hepatitis, STD, and TB Prevention: Division of Tuberculosis Elimination (DTBE).

32. O. Lubarsch, "Zur Kenntnis der auf die Samenblaschen Amyloidablagerungen," *Virchow Arch. Path. Anat.* 274 (1930): 139–145.

CHAPTER 5

Department of Neuropathology, Harvard Medical School, Boston, Massachusetts, 1909

By 1910—within three years of Alzheimer and Fischer's initial papers, Elmer Ernest Southard, Harvard professor of neuropathology, released his own paper on senile and Alzheimer's presenile dementia.

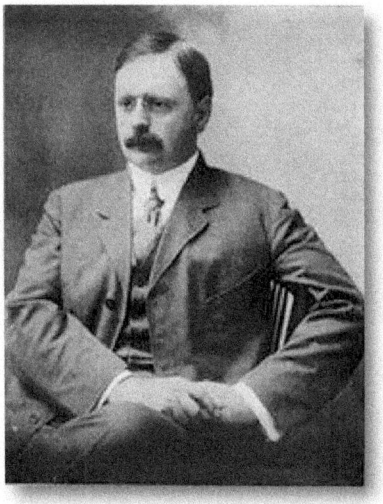

Figure 22. Dr. E. E. Southard, MD, Director of Harvard Neuropathology.

In that paper, Southard put Alzheimer and Fischer on notice that with regard to age-related senility, his autopsy of forty-two cases of what we now call Alzheimer's disease showed that the vast majority of cases had findings suggestive of tuberculosis—as a rule dormant, obsolescent, and acquired earlier in life. Furthermore, Southard reported straightforwardly that general tuberculosis could "scarcely be excluded with safety from any case" in his experience autopsying the age-related dementias.[1] In addition, Southard, an expert on the pathology of neurosyphilis, found no one-on-one linkage between neurosyphilis in either Alzheimer's or senile dementia.[2]

Kraepelin and Alzheimer's response to Southard's work was to ignore it. But Southard, regarded as the leading neuropathologist in the United States, was difficult to ignore, even for Germany's most ardent psychogenicist and psychiatric classifier-in-chief, Emil Kraepelin.

This was not the first time that Southard and Kraepelin had crossed swords. And Kraepelin would soon have more than enough of Southard, who was a major force behind the eventually successful attempt to change Kraepelin's pet popularization of "dementia praecox" back to schizophrenia.[3]

By 1904, E. E. Southard, MD, was an instructor and Bullard Professor of Neuropathology at the Harvard Medical School. Shortly after finishing his medical degree, Southard spent a brief time studying at the Senckenberg Institute at Frankfort and the University of Heidelberg in Germany.

Southard was quite blunt and to the point, regarding Kraepelin's championing of the term "dementia praecox." It meant "premature dementia," a chronic yet rapid deterioration of thought ability that usually begins in the late teens or early adulthood. Though

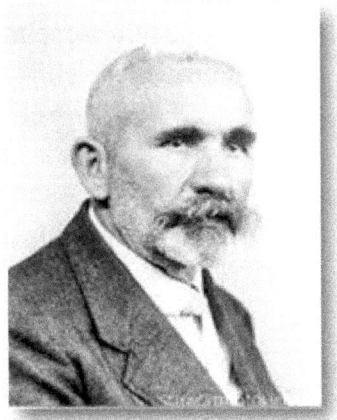

Figure 23. Emil Kraepelin.

aware that Arnold Pick first used the term in 1891, Southard was nevertheless irked by Kraepelin's continued attempts to disseminate it. He complained accordingly:

> Perhaps no more unfortunate term than *dementia praecox* has yet been devised for an important group of psychopathic patients.[4]

Although E. E. Southard subsequently would become Chairman of the Committee on Psychiatry and Neurology for the National Research Council, his research focused squarely on neuropathological studies—totally uninfluenced by psychiatry. Unlike Alzheimer, Southard had no Kraepelin to pay homage to. Kraepelin was after a brand-new illness, preferably unknown regarding cause for the sake of the financial perpetuation of his clinic. Kraepelin knew Southard's tubercular/dementia reference well, made more than familiar to him through the publications of still another one of Kraepelin's rivals, England's T. S. Clouston. In his memoirs, Kraepelin mentions Clouston's visit to Munich:

> Englishmen rarely came to visit, amongst the more well-known colleagues, Clouston came to visit.[5]

NOTES

1. E. E. Southard, "Anatomical Findings in Senile Dementia: A Diagnostic Study Bearing Especially on the Group of Cerebral Atrophies," *American Journal of Insanity* 66, no. 4 (April 1910): 673–708 p.701 p706.
2. E. E. Southard, and H. C. Solomon, Neurosypilis: Modern Systematic Diagnosis and Treatment—Presented in One Hundred and Thirty-Seven Case Histories (Boston: W. M. Leonard, 1917).
3. E. E. Southard, "Nondementia Nonpraecox: Note on the Advantages to Mental Hygiene of Extirpating a Term" in *History of Psychiatry*, Classic Text No. 72, 18, no. 4 (1919): 483–502; Los Angeles, London, New Delhi, and Singapore: Sage Publications, 2007.
4. E. E. Southard, and M. C. Jarrett, *The Kingdom of Evils: Psychiatric Social Work Presented in One Hundred Case Histories Together with a Classification of Social Divisions of Evil* (New York: Macmillan, 1922), 298–9.
5. E. Krepelin, *Memoirs* (Springer-Verlag: Berlin and New York, 1987), 270pp p136.

CHAPTER 6

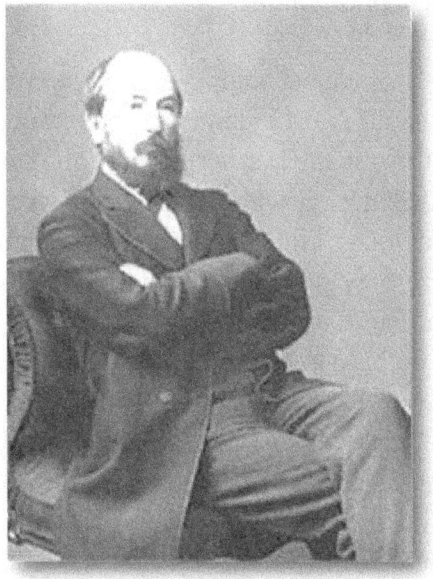

Figure 24. Sir Thomas Smith Clouston.

Clouston was "well-known," indeed. In fact, his fame at that time easily rivaled Kraepelin's. Of the two benchmark events chronicled to this day in medicine for 1883, Thomas Clouston's publication of *Clinical Lectures on Mental Diseases* sits side-by-side with Emil Kraepelin's *Compendium der Psychiatrie*.

Clouston was appointed Lecturer on Mental Diseases at the prestigious University of Edinburgh, a post he held in conjunction with his position as head of the noteworthy Royal Edinburgh Asylum. A celebrated lecturer, Clouston gained international notoriety for his explanation of the psychiatric disorders of adolescence. Publishing extensively, Clouston began with his remarkable *Clinical Lectures*, followed, later, by his more popular *Unsoundness of Mind*.[1]

Clouston, in a 463-subject autopsy-driven-study, said that tubercular patients tended to be demented before death much more than the non-tubercular. Furthermore, in the majority of cases of dementia, whether presenile or senile, Clouston found tuberculosis upon autopsy after death—provided it was looked for adequately. The only problem was, according to Clouston, that nobody, including Kraepelin and Alzheimer—and with the exception of Southard at Harvard—was adequately doing so.

Why was this? In 1917, Physician S. A. Silk of the Government Hospital for the Insane in Washington clarified why TB was not looked for in most mental institutions. Silk knew that the majority of hospitals and institutions for the "so-called" insane such as the Munich Clinic or Frankfort's Institution for the Mentally Ill still lacked special provisions for the treatment of tubercular patients. Therefore Silk concluded that "there seems quite a reluctance on the part of the medical staffs to pronounce their patients tubercular, which was possibly due to the unjust opinion among the laity that tuberculosis occurring in mental asylums is due to unsanitary conditions of the hospital or improper care of the patients."[2] In most institutions, he pointed out, no case was even considered tuberculous unless a positive sputum for tuberculosis was obtained, which was often falsely negative, if it was tested for at all—"leaving many tuberculous cases undiagnosed."[2]

In another study of 282 cases, Clouston[3] addressed just what S. A. Silk was referring to, insisting that tubercular psychiatric disease had nothing to do with asylum conditions because it was often present in newly confined cases. Nor, said Clouston, did long-term confinement for a condition like age-related dementia lend itself more to tuberculosis than any other disease that afflicted humans. In addition, he cautioned that in up to one-third of cases in the demented and mentally afflicted, their tuberculosis could be entirely latent and asymptomatic, again leading to tuberculosis's gross underestimation, both in mental institutions and among the demented.

Actually, Thomas Clouston was proving to be an annoying thorn in Emil Kraepelin's side on several levels. Clouston first coined the term "adolescent insanity" in 1873 for what Emil Kraepelin now insisted was dementia praecox. Clouston maintained that it was a serious condition from which 30 percent of victims wound up with a more serious "secondary dementia." This subset of Clouston's patients seemed in accord with Bleuler, who advanced the theory that Kraepelin's so-called "dementia praecox" of adolescence and certain senile dementias were identical.

This was the last thing Emil Kraepelin wanted to hear. Although the word "dementia" was part of his "dementia praecox," Kraepelin did not want it to be thought of in any way as a take-off point leading to senile dementia. To this end, Kraepelin rarely used the term "senile dementia" or "presenile Alzheimer's dementia" to refer to the end state of his dementia praecox (schizophrenia).

Clouston knew all about the arbitrariness of Kraepelin's classifications, as well as Kraepelin's fondness for borrowing the terminology and concepts of others. Kraepelin had lifted his entire idea for a comprehensive psychiatric classification system directly from the writings of fellow German psychiatrist Karl Kahlbaum. So when Kraepelin used the term "dementia praecox" for what Clouston had already labeled "adolescent or developmental insanity" without specifically mentioning Clouston, Clouston felt angry, usurped, and slighted:

> Since I first used the term in 1873 and described its general characteristics, it has become generally accepted by writers in psychiatry. Lately, however, Kraepelin has taken the term *dementia praecox* and applied it to practically my whole group of adolescent cases, making it cover the curable and incurable. I strongly object...[4]

Just as annoying, from Kraepelin's viewpoint, was Clouston's finding that most of the people who died of tuberculosis in mental institutions were demented and that Clouston's third stage of tubercular dementia in effect mirrored the symptoms of end-stage Alzheimer's, leading to "the abolition of mind in all its forms, of senile dementia."[1]

To Emil Kraepelin, this was a high-stakes conflict, and Kraepelin knew that very well. At that point, half of the deaths in the young-aged population that dementia praecox visited were from TB, which was repeatedly being linked to dementia praecox/schizophrenia in the literature of that day. If there was a direct infectious continuum involving the evolution of dementia praecox/schizophrenia to Alzheimer's presenile dementia and then on to senile dementia itself, then two of Kraepelin's cherished categories—praecox and Alzheimer's disease—were in jeopardy. Indeed the term "Alzheimer's disease" would be superfluous, a mere pit stop as dementia praecox evolved in some people toward senile dementia. Therefore, Kraepelin would go to any and all extremes to downplay such a linkage, including his sleight of hand of leaving out some of the actual contents in Auguste Deter's chart. Clearly Deter's postmortem included findings included tangles, Fischer's plaques, and arteriosclerotic changes in her brain—accompanied by Alzheimer's earlier clinical mention of her hallucinations and delusions. Perusini could not confirm the atherosclerotic changes at autopsy. But in his own announcement, Kraepelin left out Deter's "hallucinations" and "delusions" that Alzheimer previously charted.[5]

This left the historic question of why Kraepelin would do this. Kraepelin was already on record as saying that delusions and hallucinations were primary symptoms in his dementia praecox (schizophrenia)—concepts that are still very much with us. Therefore, Alzheimer's charting of Deter's delusions and hallucinations left Kraepelin in the uncomfortable position of having to explain why Alzheimer was picking up symptoms in Alzheimer's disease that he had already declared primary to schizophrenia (dementia praecox).

Kraepelin's solution was to sidestep the issue altogether, leaving out mention of Deter's delusions and hallucinations. In the same manner, Kraepelin would neglect to mention that Beljahow discussed the original pathology underlying Alzheimer's disease as early as 1887, followed by Fuller, Redlich, Leri, and Oskar Fischer.

But, as is often the case, covering up certain facts would not be adequate to cover up others. The ineradicable evidence is that in his first classical 1897 study, Alzheimer[6] showed that patients with schizophrenia (dementia praecox) also exhibited increased neurofibrillary tangles and neuritic plaques, albeit to a lesser degree. In fact, the rates of dementia in those aging individuals with a history of schizophrenia are twice that of non-schizophrenic patients.[7]

Add to this Kraepelin's own statement, "The fatal termination of the catatonic cases [of dementia praecox or schizophrenia] usually occurs as the result of some intercurrent disease, of which tuberculosis is the most prominent"[8], and you will understand why Emil Kraepelin would take any measure at his disposal to distance his newly minted "Alzheimer's disease" from schizophrenia, its attending dementia, and the then-mushrooming literature attributing schizophrenia to a tubercular cause.

Enter the historic debate regarding tuberculosis, schizophrenia, and the dementias…

NOTES

1. T. S. Clouston, *Unsoundness of Mind* (New York: E. F. Dutton and Co., 1911).
2. S. A. Silk, "The Physical Changes Observed in Pulmonary Tuberculosis and Its Relation to Insanity," *Medical Record* 92, no. 23 (December 8, 1917), 976.
3. T.S. Clouston, "The Connection between Tuberculosis and Insanity" *Journal of Mental Science*. The Association of Medical Officers of Asylums and Hospitals for the Insane Publisher, No. 45 (April, 1863)
4. T. S. Clouston, *Clinical Lectures on Mental Diseases*, 6th edition (London: Churchill, 1904).
5. G. E. Berrios, "Alzheimer's Disease: A Conceptual History," *International Journal of Geriatric Psychiatry* 5, no. 6 (1990) 355–65].
6. A. Alzheimer, "Beitrage zur Pathologischen Anatomie der Hirnrinde und zur Anatomischen Grundlage der Psychosen," *Mschr. Psychiat. Neurol.* 2 (1897):82–112.
7. H. C. Hendrie, W. Tu, R. Tabbey, C. E. Purnell, R. J. Ambuehl, and C. M. Callahan, "Health Outcomes and Cost of Care Among Older Adults with Schizophrenia: A Ten-Year Study Using Medical Records across the Continuum of Care," *The American Journal of Geriatric Psychiatry* 22, no. 5 (May 2014): 427–36.
8. A. R. Diefendorf, "Clinical Psychiatry for Students and Physicians" adapted from the 7th German edition of *Kraepelin's Lehrbuch der Psychiatrie*, new edition, revised and augmented (New York and London: The Macmillan Company, 1912), 256–7.

CHAPTER 7

Psychiatric and Mental Asylums on the European and American Continents, Late Nineteenth Century and Early Twentieth Century

Despite the fact that Kraepelin left out the fact that Auguste Deter, the first Alzheimer's disease patient had "hallucinations" and "delusions," she did, as Alzheimer himself previously charted.

Almost unheard of in the medical literature before 1800, chronic delusions and hallucinations—like hearing voices—became common in asylum admissions. At the same time, Clouston, by 1892, was documenting hallucinations (mainly auditory) and delusions with regularity in mental illness as a result of a killer pandemic of tuberculosis prevalent at the time.[1] Historians like Edward Hare and Robert Wilkins, among others, point out that it was only then that schizophrenia, a mental disease often with such hallucinations and delusions, was really even mentioned, representing no small part of the nineteenth-century flare-up of psychiatric admissions.[2,3]

Johann Greding's large series found[4] pulmonary tuberculosis in 50 percent of mental patients with convulsive disorders. Because seizures were not uncommon in the course of schizophrenia, schizophrenics seemed well represented.

Greding wasn't alone.

Barr talked about the relationship between tuberculosis and mental defectiveness, including dementia, at the Sixth International Tuberculosis Congress held in Washington in 1908.[5] Jacques Moreau believed that epilepsy and the convulsive disorders were largely derived from tuberculosis, as did his colleague, Anglade. This was fifteen years after Gheorghe Marinescu and Paul Blocq, while working in the Salpêtrière in Paris, described neuritic plaque deposits in the brains of elderly patients with epilepsy. Anglade saw a direct path toward becoming mentally defective through the sclerotic brain changes caused by the disease.[6] Such sclerosis was not only written up in Redlich's and Leri's findings of senile plaque as "miliary sclerosis," but Hektoen found that it was a characteristic vascular end-stage change for cerebral tuberculosis.

Subsequently, Baruk discovered that when either the proteins extracted from tuberculosis, or the spinal fluid taken from schizophrenics was introduced into healthy animals, a condition occurred in which the body and its functions seemed frozen in time, called "catalepsy," not only associated with one form of schizophrenia but with epilepsy itself.[7] Kraepelin had mentioned the tendency that TB had to possibly result in such schizophrenic catalepsy, but Baruk introduced the thought that the mechanism through which this might happen could be the tuberculoproteins from systemic foci, an "allergic" reaction to the protein itself, because tuberculous bacilli were not always found. Whereas Kraepelin would emphasize TB as the usual origin of just one type of dementia praecox/schizophrenia, others disagreed.

This set the stage for prominent Viennese pathologist Ernst Lowenstein, who decided to take things a step further. Having developed a potato-flour-and-egg-based tuberculosis growth medium, still very much with us, Lowenstein set about to prove that TB could be cultured from the blood of patients with a number of medical conditions of unknown cause, including "schizophrenia," his primary target.[8]

D'Hollander,[9] Coste,[10] and Ciarla[11] independently confirmed Lowenstein's positive tubercular blood cultures for schizophrenia. Similarly, Claude,[12] Puca,[13] Toulouse,[14] Couderc,[15] and Stefan[16] also indirectly confirmed Lowenstein's tubercular schizophrenic cause—not by targeting the tuberculosis's bacillus itself, but its forms, which are much harder to stain and culture, yet commoner, viral-like, and cell-wall-deficient. These were the forms Fontes[17] described in 1910, when Alzheimer and Fischer were working on senile dementia.

To all of these researchers of dementia praecox, the view that a filter-passing "virus" coming from the tubercular disease decimating Europe and then the United States seemed more tenable then the conventional filterable virus theory circulating at that time.[18] Yet despite these nine independent confirmative studies finding TB in the blood of schizophrenics, other studies appeared that could not confirm their results, perhaps as a result of inadequate laboratory technique.

Unshaken, and in answer to these negative studies, Weeber,[19] Welajah,[20] Melgar,[21] and Lowenstein[22] himself again found tuberculosis in the blood of schizophrenic patients in studies that have remained unaddressed to this day.

When Auguste Deter died, Clouston noted, she was examined by two of Alzheimer's colleagues, who recorded the cause of death in her medical file as follows:

> During the morning *exitus letalis*; cause of death: infection in the blood [septicemia] due to decubitus; anatomical diagnosis: moderate hydrocephalus (external internal); cerebral atrophy; arteriosclerosis of the small cerebral blood vessels; (?); pneumonia of both inferior lobes; nephritis.[23]

Deter therefore had moderate hydrocephalus.

As far back as 1769, Scotsman Robert Whytt, reporting on approximately twenty cases, described the localization of tuberculosis in the meninges, membranes that cover the brain and spinal cord.[24] Realizing that the localization of tuberculosis there was often associated with mental disturbances, Whytt noticed not only small masses called "tubercles" in the brain tissue but hydrocephalus, an excess of "water in the brain."

Because hydrocephalus is a medical condition in which there is an abnormal accumulation of cerebrospinal fluid in the ventricles, or deep cavities, in the brain, this may cause increased intracranial pressure inside the skull, with possible progressive enlargement of the head, seizures, or mental disability. By 1911 and before, hydrocephalus and tuberculosis[25] had become so intertwined that medical experts by the end of the nineteenth century (Alzheimer first saw Auguste Deter just after this) considered acute hydrocephalus as just another name for tuberculous meningitis.

Had the parallels between neurotuberculosis and Alzheimer's disease ended with their penchant for both causing hydrocephalus, it would be remarkable and little else. But such similarities went far beyond that and included the fact that Alzheimer's and tuberculosis share a common site of origin: the base of the brain.

This predisposition for tuberculosis to affect the base or bottom of the brain makes its initial attack unlike any other intracranial infection—including dementia caused by neurosyphilis, where the chief pathological changes are found in the substance of the cerebral hemispheres. With time, it became obvious that Alzheimer's genesis, more often than not, also first affected brain structures close to, or at the base (or bottom) of the brain. By the same token, since 1901, Vigouroux's study[26] of a dying schizophrenic revealed the all too familiar basilar pathology of tuberculosis at the bottom of the brain, a location of early attack that appears in countless studies, including those of Kirman[27], Marchand.[28] and on to the present day.

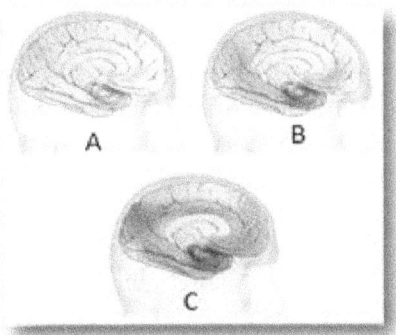

Figure 25. Plaques and tangles in Alzheimer's (shown in the shaded areas inside the cranium) tend to spread through the cortex in a predictable pattern as Alzheimer's disease progresses. The rate of progression varies greatly. Note that the disease begins (A) toward the base or bottom of the brain, fanning out from that point across the convexity of the cortex (B and C).

One of the structures near the base, or bottom, of the brain is the hippocampus, critical to Alzheimer's neuropathology. If the surface of the cerebral hemispheres is regarded as a sphere with a broad-based indentation on its bottom, then one of the structures that lines the edge of this hollow depression is the hippocampus.

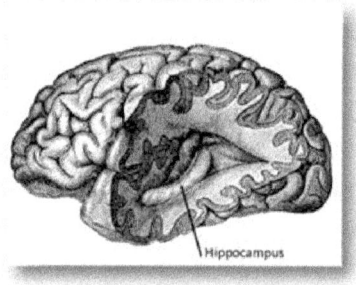

Figure 26. The human hippocampus. Although the gross visual examination of the Alzheimer's brain is not diagnostic, a typical early symmetric pattern of cortical atrophy predominantly affects the human brain's medial temporal lobes. One side of a lobe has been cut away here to show its underlying hippocampus.

The hippocampal region, located in the medial temporal lobe, is responsible for storing new information and memory formation. It is affected early and often in Alzheimer's.

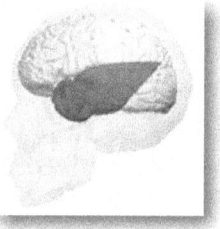

Figure 27. The medial temporal lobe, which here assumes the shape of an arrowhead in the middle of this picture—a region critical for memory.

Besides, the hippocampal region the medial temporal lobe also consists of structures that are vital for long-term memory. The hippocampus is crucially important for memory formation, but its surrounding medial temporal cortex is currently theorized to be critical for memory storage.[29]

Prominent atrophy, or wasting away, of this memory region is usually observed early on in both Alzheimer's and tuberculosis. Pando[30] and others have documented that in a full-scale tubercular attack on the same region, neurons in the hippocampal area showed significant damage, eaten away through necrosis and extensive gliosis. Certainly, thought Pando, the possibility of such tubercular targeting of the hippocampal area should be considered in memory or cognitive disturbance.

Furthermore, the middle cerebral artery supplies most of the blood to the temporal-lobe origins of Alzheimer's.

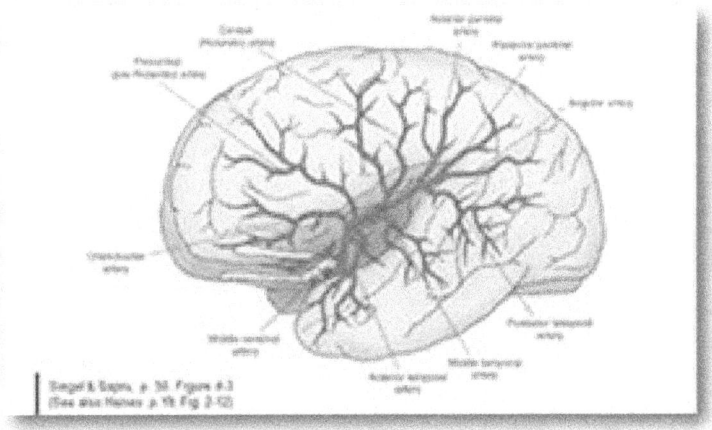

Figure 28: The middle cerebral artery and its branches.

Something was being brought into the Alzheimer's brain through the middle cerebral artery, blood-borne and infectious enough to spread—the same middle cerebral artery (MCA) that together with its branches are the most common vessels in the brain infected by neurotuberculosis.[31] Although many other vessels in the brain can be diseased, the vessel that is infected by cerebral tuberculosis most commonly is this MCA and its branches, the favored portal of entry. It is precisely because of such preferred middle cerebral artery transport that tubercles most frequently land first and are housed in the lateral and medial aspects of the temporal lobes—the same medial temporal lobe that accommodates the early instigations of Alzheimer's disease. There Alzheimer's begins to weave its web of amyloid plaque, neurofibrillary tangles, and ischemic infarcts ("strokes") typically found on autopsy in approximately 20 percent of Alzheimer's victims.[32]

NOTES

1. T. S. Clouston, "Phthisical Insanity," in *History of Psychiatry* 64, no. 4 (December 2005): 479–95.
2. E. Hare, "Was Insanity on the Increase?" *British Medical Journal* 142 (1983): 439–45.
3. R. Wilkins, "Hallucinations in Children and Teenagers Admitted to Bethlem Royal Hospital in the Nineteenth Century and Their Possible Relevance to the Incidence of Schizophrenia," *Journal of Child Psychology and Psychiatry* 28 (1987): 569–80.
4. J. Greding, *Sammtliche Medicinische Schriften*, C. W. Greding, Ed. Greiz, and Henning (eds.) (1790): vol. I: 277–350; vol. II: 145–62, 327–33.
5. M. W. Barr, "The relationship between Tuberculosis and Mental Defect," Sixth *International Congress on Tuberculosis*, Washington, 1908; Philadelphia, 1908, 88.
6. Anglade and Jacquin, "Heredo-Tuberculose et Idioties Congenitales," *Encephale* 1 (1907): 136–57.
7. H. Baruk, *Psychiatrie. Medicale, Physiologique et Experimental* (Paris: Masson et Cie. 1938)
8. E. Lowenstein, "Das Vorkommen der Tuberkelbazillamie bei verschiedenen Krankheiten," *Munch. Med. Wschr.* 78 (1931): 261–63.
9. F. D'Hollander, "Rouvroy Recherches Experimentales Sur la Demence Precoce," *C. R. Soc. Biol.* 110 (1932): 570–2.
10. F. Coste, et al., "Constatations Experimentales Concernant L'etiologie Tuberculeuse de Certaines Demences Precoces," *Bull. Acad. Med.*, 109 (1933): 760–4.
11. E. Ciarla and G. C. Torri, "Tentativi di Cultura del Bacillo Tubercular su Terreno di Lowenstein da Sangue e

Liquid Cefalorachidiano di Schizofrenici e di Altri Malati Mentali,"*Boll Ist Sieroter Milan*14 (1935): 1031–36.

12. H. Claude and F. Coste, "Sur Les Relations de la Tuberculose et de la Demence Precoce," *C. R. Soc. Biol.* 116 (1934): 1356–9.

13. A. Puca, "Sur la Mise en Evidence de Ganules Acido-Resistants et de Bacillus Dans Les Organs de Cobayes Inocules Avec le Liquid Cephalorachidien de Dements Precoces," *C. R. Soc. Biol.* 111 (1932): 258–60.

14. E. Toulouse, et al., "Ultra-Virus Tuberculeux et Demence Precoce," *Ann. Med.-Psychol.* 2 (1932): 474–86.

15. L. Couderc, "La Démence Precoce Peut-Elle etre Virus Neurotrope de Nature Tuberculeuse," *Ann. med.-psychol.,* 2 (1932): 496–9.

16. H. Stefan, "loserkuloser Charakter und Tuberkulose Psychose. Ein Fall Einer Syptomatischen Psychose, Verursacht Durch das Tuberkulose Virus," *Arch. Psychiat. Nervenkr.* 100 (1933): 352–63.

17. A. Fontes, "Bemerkungen Ueber Die Tuberculoese Infection und ihr Virus, *Mem Instit Oswaldo Crus* 2 (1910): 141–6.

18. E. Hare in *Research on the Viral Hypothesis of Mental Disorders: Advances in Biological Psychiatry*, vol. 12, P. V. Morozov (ed.) (Karger: Basle, 1983), 52–75.

19. R. Weeber, "Ueber Blutund Liquorbazillose," *Wien. Med. Wschr.* 87 (1937): 285–6.

20. M. H. Welajah, "Role Played by Filterable Viruses in the Causation of Insanity," *Journal of the Egyptian Medical Association* 23 (1940): 178–9.

21. R. Melger, "Tuberculosis y Psicosis," *Rev. Asoc. Med. Argent.* 57 (1943): 1061–4.

22. E. Lowenstein, "Tubercle Bacilli in Spinal Fluid," *Journal of Nervous and Mental Disease* 101 (1945): 576–82.
23. K. Maurer, S. Volk, and H. Gerbaldo, "Auguste D and Alzheimer's Disease," *Lancet* 349 (1997): 1546–49.
24. R. Whytt, *Observation on the Dropsy of the Brain* (Edinburgh, 1768).
25. Encyclopedia Britannica, edited by H. Chisholm (London: Cambridge University Press, 1911). At that time, the diagnosis of acute hydrocephalus was so commonly associated with tuberculous meningitis that the terms were used interchangeably.
26. A. Vigouroux, "Meningite Tuberculeuse a Forme Melancolique," *Ann. Med.-Psychol.* 2 (1901): 309–14.
27. B. H. Kirman, "Mental Symptoms in Tuberculous Meningitis," *British Journal of Tuberculosis*, 37 (1943): 63–8.
28. L. Marchand and J. deAjuriaguerra, "De la Meningite Tuberculeuse Chez L'adult; Ses Forms Psychiques," *Progr. Med.* 73 (1945): 447–51.
29. Kosslyn Smith, *Cognitive Psychology: Mind and Brain* (New Jersey: Prentice Hall, 2007), 21, 194–9, 349.
30. R. H. Pando, D. Aguilar, I. Cohen, M. Guerrero, W. Ribon, et al., "Model Systems: Specific Bacterial Genotypes of *Mycobacterium tuberculosis* Cause Extensive Dissemination and Brain Infection in an Experimental Model," *Tuberculosis* 90 (2010): 268–77.
31. P. Subramanian, "Bacteria and Bacterial Diseases in Walsh and Hoyt's Clinical Neuro-Ophthalmology," Degenerative and Metabolic Diseases, 6th ed., vol. 3 (2005):2690.
32. D. P. Perl, "Neuropathology of Alzheimer's Disease," *Mount Sinai Journal of Medicine* 77 (2010): 32–42.

CHAPTER 8

Anatomie Laboratorium, Nervenklinik, Department of Clinical Psychiatry, University of Munich, Germany, 1910

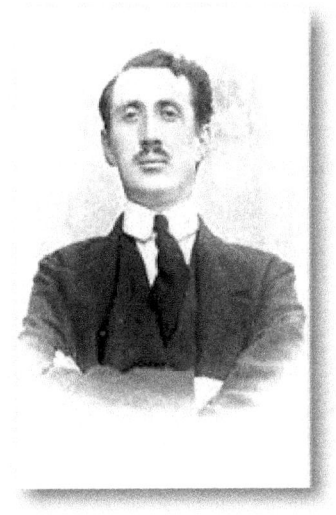

Figure 29. Gaetano Perusini, 1910.

Showing all the assurance of a favored son, Alzheimer's young workhorse, Gaetano Perusini, proceeded to autopsy the four cases Alzheimer assigned to him, the first of which was the brain of Auguste Deter. Perusini was bright. Perusini was intuitive. In addition, Perusini spoke fluent German. But Perusini was also rather young and clinically unseasoned, having graduated from the School of Medicine of the Catholic University in Rome and then having specialized mainly in the "endemic cretinism" prevalent in northern Italy — Tabes Dorsalis of syphilitic origin, and Friedreich's condition.[1] He would work in Alzheimer's laboratory until 1912 and die within three years of his departure, a young life cut short while trying to save a fellow soldier during World War 1. Gaetano Perusini was thirty-six when he died, ironically just one week before Alois Alzheimer died of an unknown chronic disease at fifty-one—a disease that manifested itself in heart and kidney complications. Kraepelin would later say that Alzheimer explained his own condition as an infectious angina with nephritic kidney disease and inflammation of the joints.[2] Others would more specifically add that Alzheimer died of cardiac failure secondary to infectious endocarditis, first called "infectious" by 1878 Edwin Klebs in Germany, who believed all cases of endocarditis were infectious in origin.

When Alzheimer published the fourth volume of his book emphasizing abnormal tissue in the cerebral cortex of brains with mental disease, one of its chapters was titled "The Perusini Cases." Perusini helped Alzheimer define Alzheimer's disease so much that some, to this day, call it "la malattia di Alzheimer-Perusini"…the disease of Alzheimer-Perusini.[3]

One of the Alzheimer's autopsies Perusini performed was on a syphilitic. But that patient also had apical lung scarring from pulmonary tuberculosis. The other three patients assigned to him did not have syphilis. Perusini knew that with regard to syphilis being behind Alzheimer's disease that Alzheimer, as well as Oskar Fischer of Prague, never gave even a hint or implication that syphilis was exclusively or largely behind Alzheimer's. Perusini indicated that in syphilis, "the brain usually lacks the described plaques and ganglion cell alterations"—yet it was in this case of syphilis along with lung scarring from a tubercular attack that Perusini saw just such plaques and tangles. Perusini called the tubercular lung lesion "old" yet simultaneously left the door open in general to an "old" cause for his Alzheimer's patients. He noted that "all observations in the cerebral cortex [including plaques and tangles] and particularly in the glia indicate with certainty that we are dealing with an old pathological process that advances over the course of years."

Perusini understood that coworker and compatriot Francesco leaned toward syphilis as the main cause of Alzheimer's disease, but Perusini was certain that Bonfigliio was wrong. And Perusini would now move to make this clear in a detailed review of three out of four Alzheimer's autopsy victims—a study with seventy-nine figures published in 1910.[4]

In all four cases, Gaetano Perusini noticed plaque formation side-by-side with neurofibrillary tangle changes and is certain that there was a connection between the formation of the plaques and the tangles. In fact, to Perusini, the formation of plaques with fibrillary tangles was an essential finding regarding Alzheimer's disease. Not so for Oskar Fischer, who found tangles only in approximately 20 percent of his age-related senile dementia autopsies—a disorder Fischer refused to differentiate from Alzheimer's "presenile" disease. Indeed, Fischer pointed out, neurofibrillary tangles did not exist in Alzheimer's second patient. Simchowicz was first to use the term "senile plaque." The term "plaque," however, has not historically been reserved for either Alzheimer's disease or senile dementia. As far back as 1830, Papavoine[5] described the tubercles of tuberculosis as "plaques" and granulations in the brain's pia mater (see fig. 30 below), the very area that Perusini now saw major Alzheimer's alterations in.

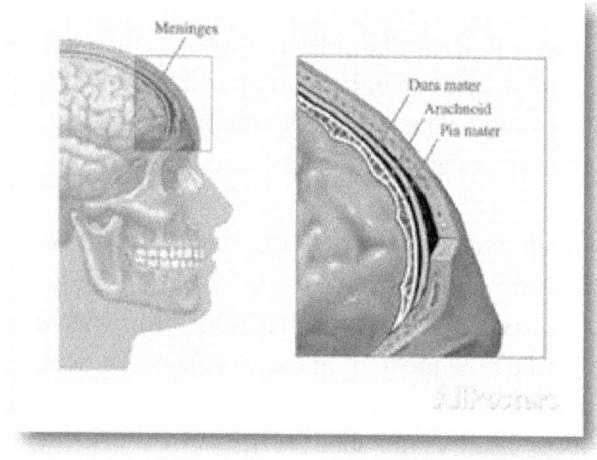

Figure 30. The pia mater, or "pia," which is the innermost of the three coverings of the brain called the "meninges." The pia mater, as shown above, firmly adheres to the surface of the brain and spinal cord. It is a very thin membrane but highly vascular and filled with small blood vessels.

Papavoine was not the first to study the pia with regard to tuberculosis. Previously, Rindfleisch[6] closely followed the histology of miliary tubercles in the pia, finding the larger arteries to be the seat of unilateral swelling, while the smaller arteries presented spindle-shaped thickenings—all originating in the adventitia of blood vessels (see fig. 31). Fischer described similar spindle-shaped thickenings of nerve fibers terminating with club forms in plaques.

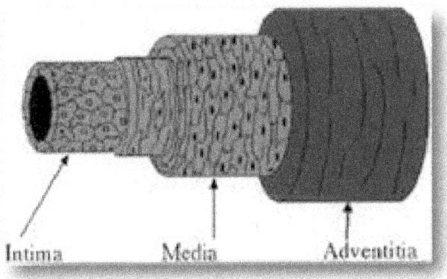

Figure 31. The layers of an artery. Its adventitia is on the outside, the external coating of a blood vessel. The adventia is a tough layer consisting mainly of collagen fibers that act supportively. Perusini found thickening of the Alzheimer's adventia. Hektoen explained that tubercle bacilli, carried by the blood, were also localized in the arterial adventitia. In fact, "In cerebral arteries only the adventitia is usually involved," Hektoen wrote.

To Barlow,[7] such infiltration of the pia with cerebral tuberculosis could also lead to the classic Alzheimer's degeneration reported by Fischer and Alzheimer of both the central mass of nerve fibers (axis-cylinders) and ganglion cells—leading, at times, to neurofibrillary tangles. By 1915, Sir William Osler[8] spoke of the "plaque" of focal tuberculous meningoencephalitis, usually situated on the surface of one of the cerebral hemispheres and less often elsewhere. Although of meningeal origin, Osler said, the involvement of cortical tissue from such tubercular plaque was inevitable.

In his summary, Perusini stressed that fiber alterations and plaque formation were limited to the cerebral cortex. Chief pathologist of Johns Hopkins, Arnold Rich, talked about small, focal, tubercular plaques ranging from one or two millimeters to a centimeter in size on the meningeal lining or cerebral cortex of the brain. Rich mentioned that although such plaque was repeatedly observed in the literature on tuberculosis, its character was not yet sufficiently appreciated. Such plaque, Rich added, depending on its location and the consequent pressure conditions under which it developed, commonly appeared as irregular, flattened, plaque-like masses.[9]

Gaetano Perusini continued to summarize his Alzheimer's findings:

> A further common finding in all three cases [that were not syphilitic] concerning the blood vessels is the thickened appearance of the adventitia, earlier described. This adventitial enlargement was common to both small and large blood vessels of the brain: at times, presented as quite strange thickenings, occasionally only involving one side of the blood vessel. At times this gave a half moon appearance in the Van Gieson preparation while in others, the blood vessel sometimes appears as a thick lumen-less [closed] red ring so that it could be confused with amyloid bodies...[2]

Approximately two and a half decades before this, Guarneri[10] studied the histological changes in twelve cases of tuberculous meningitis, seeing similar thickened adventitia, with the same strange semilunar half-moon thickenings that Perusini mentions, occasionally involving one side of the blood vessel. And fourteen years before Perusini, Hektoen,[11] in the Rockefeller *Journal of Experimental Pathology*, saw similar vascular changes in cerebral tuberculosis "in the form of a homogeneous ring which stains…bright red with Van Gieson's stain" and with particular thickening, once again, of the adventitia.

So according to Hektoen, Perusini's findings of thickening of the Alzheimer's adventia simulate what happens when tubercle bacilli, carried by the blood, are localized in the arterial adventitia. In fact, "In cerebral arteries only the adventitia is usually involved," Hektoen wrote. He added, "All authors emphasize the prominent part played by the adventitia in the formation of the tubercles and more diffuse infiltrations in tuberculous meningitis.[11] This, Hektoen said, was because It was in the lymph spaces in this adventitial layer of the arterial wall that the tubercle bacilli appeared to find the most favorable conditions for rapid growth.

Perusini's summary of tissue changes generally found in Alzheimer's continued to mirror Hektoen's findings on tubercular changes involving the brain. When Perusini talked about the ability of Alzheimer's to make changes in the intima of pial arteries as well as the arterial adventitia, Hektoen made this statement:

> The general conclusion is consequently warranted that in tuberculous meningitis of bloodborne infection an unexpectedly frequent and significant localization of the bacilli occurs upon the intima of pial arteries in addition to that in the arterial adventitia.[11]

Perusini also noted that plaque and tangle formation in all four of his cases of Alzheimer's were limited to the cerebral cortex, even in the one case with severe spinal-cord involvement.

Hektoen observed that tuberculosis, with time, also preferred to attack the cerebral cortex.

Perusini remarked that it was probable that the deeply "fuchsinophilic" nucleus-poor thickenings of the adventitia he saw in Alzheimer's would have been included—a few years earlier—in the concept of "hyaline degeneration." But a year after Gaetano Perusini's publication, investigators Bruno Bandelier and Otto Roepke not only reported that TB meningitis "affects constantly the cerebral cortex"; they reported how it creates the same "hyaline degeneration" Perusini was referring to. "Hyaline degeneration" was the term that both Guarnieri and Ludvig Hektoen used to describe the end-stage attack on a tubercular blood vessel. Indeed, Guarnieri[10] after studying the histological changes in twelve cases of tuberculous meningitis—besides documenting adventitial changes and the infiltration of the disease into nerves—specifically mentioned hyaline degeneration of a vessel as the end result of cerebral tuberculosis. In addition, Perusini's description of "fuchsinophilic" thickenings in the adventitia in no way precludes that such thickenings were not the result of intracellular, acid-fast tubercular-like bacilli.[12]

Common to both Perusini's and Alzheimer's papers is the mention of widespread lipid or fat accumulation in the Alzheimer's brain. Perusini wrote the following about the widespread lipid (also called lipoid) he saw during the Auguste Deter autopsy:

> Cerebral cortex: fat preparations (Osmium stain, Herxheimer method) show a large quantity of lipoid substance widely distributed in all areas of the cerebral convolutions. It is found in the ganglion cells,

glial cells, and also in the cells of the vascular sheath. There is no focal accumulation of this substance. It is also abundantly found around the vessels of the cerebral cortex and the spinal cord and in various convolutions.[3, p.85]

Perusini summarized his autopsy findings that he saw "massive accumulation of lipoid substances in the ganglion cells, in the glia and vessels."[3, p.125] Similar references to fat or lipid accumulation, but from cerebral tuberculosis, come from the writings of Ursula F. Rowlatt,[13] who not only saw fatty breakdown products within the cortical ribbon but also fat in either compound granular fatty pigments or lying loose as droplets or crystals at brain autopsy.

Senile brain plaque is associated with diffuse nerve-cell changes, including some degree of atrophy and an accumulation of fatty (lipoid) pigment, which can fill the basal or bottom portions of such senile plaque to a greater or lesser degree with yellow lipoid material. Such yellow plaque fatty material is present in the form of granules of "lipofuscin," which appears as brown granules. Lipofuscin increases with age, but besides its presence with aging—and much greater presence with senile dementia and senile brain plaque—lipofuscin can also accumulate in chronic wasting diseases such as tuberculosis or cerebral tuberculosis. In addition, lipofuscin can be stained with acid fuchsin in the same acid-fast method used for *Mycobacterium tuberculosis*.[14]

The high lipid content present in tuberculous is well known. *M. tuberculosis* is unique among bacterial pathogens in that it displays a wide array of complex lipids and lipoglycans on its cell surface.[15] The fatty degeneration and fat dispersal of tubercular attack on body or brain was long ago identified as a premier feature of TB's pathology, which even included pigments seen under a low-power microscope that were linked to minute globules of fat.[16] In other cases, a tendency toward tubercular hyaline formation was noted. Toxic mycobacterial lipids are released from macrophages infected by TB either inside or outside of the brain. Such lipid dispersal is believed to expand the microbes' influence beyond the immediate confines of its host cells.[17]

Just months earlier, Perusini saw Kraepelin shaken when the American professor, Southard, now at Harvard, published autopsy-based linkage of active or dormant TB to Alzheimer's. By all indications, E. E. Southard was one of the most remarkable physicians in early twentieth-century medicine. In fact, Southard[18] had reported that general systemic tuberculosis could "scarcely be excluded with safety from any case" of age-related dementia or Alzheimer's disease.

The single worst disease present in European cities was tuberculosis, and even by 1800, it was understood that no other disease was as common or as deadly. Yet Perusini knew that Alzheimer and Kraepelin both paid little attention to the one disease except for syphilis that could possibly account for the sudden rise in age-related dementias. Rather, through Alzheimer, Kraepelin made certain that scientists, including those at his Munich Clinic, were told not to look toward well-known disease as being behind this new disease. But what was really the reason for the avoidance of even the mention of cerebral tuberculosis as a possible contributor to the age-related dementias? The reason was that just as individuals and families where penalized for having the disease, so too were mental institutions, which admitted harboring more than a modest number of such tubercular cases.

Koch himself had actually used tubercles from the brain of humans who had died of bloodborne miliary (millet-seed-like), tuberculosis to inoculate his guinea pigs with...mentioning that his usage of the term "miliary tuberculosis" was for a common yet "acute, systemic form of the disease."[19] Koch first presented this finding at a meeting of the Physiological Society of Berlin on March 24, 1882. Many of the early investigators of Alzheimer's, including Oskar Fischer, spoke of a tuberculosis-like "miliary necrosis" of neurofibrils or a miliary distribution of affected areas as a common change of the cerebral cortex in senile or presenile dementia.

Yet again, when it came to drawing from a history of studies implicating the resemblance of presenile Alzheimer's dementia to tuberculosis, Perusini, Alzheimer, and Kraepelin remained noticeably mute.

NOTES

1. M. Marta and M. Pomponi, "Il Ruolo di Perusini Nella Definizione del Morbo di Alzheimer," *Kos.* 77 (1992): 39–41.
2. A. Tagarelli, A. Piro, G. Tagarelli, P. Lagonia, and A. Quattrone, "Alois Alzheimer: A Hundred Years after the Discovery of the Eponymous Disorder," *International Journal of Biomedical Science* 2, no. 2 (June 2006): 198.
3. B. Braun, M. Stadlober-Degwerth, and H. Kluemann, "Alzheimer–Perusini Disease: The One-Hundredth Anniversary of Gaetano Perusini's Publication," *Nervenarzt* 82, no. 3 (March 2011): 363–6, 368–9.
4. G. Perusini, *Histology and Clinical Findings of Some Psychiatric Diseases of Older People in Histologische und histopathologishe Arbeiten*, vol. III, F. Nissl and A. Alzheimer (eds.) (Jena, Germany: Gustav Fischer, 1910), 297–351, in *The Early Story of Alzheimer's Disease* (Katherine Bick, Luigi Amaducci, and Giancarlo Pepeu, eds.) (Padova: Liviana Press, 1987): 82–128.
5. Louis-Nicolas Papavoine, "Propositions Sur Les Tubercules Considérés Spécialement Chez le Enfans," dissertation no. 86, v. 231, 1830, Paris.
6. Rindfleisch, "Der Miliare Tuberkel," *Virchow's Arch.* XXIV (1862): 571.
7. T. Barlow, *Tuberculous Meningitis in a System of Medicine by Many Writers*, edited by Thomas Clifford Allbutt, vol. VIII (New York: The Macmillan Company, 1899), 466–91.
8. W. Osler and T. McCrae, *Modern Medicine: Its Theory and Practice*, vol. V: *Diseases of the Nervous System*, 2nd edition (Philadelphia and New York: Lea & Febiger, 1915), 319.
9. A. R. Rich, *The Pathogenesis of Tuberculosis* (Springfield, Illinois: Chas. C. Thomas, 1946).
10. G. Guarnieri, "Note Istologiche Sulla Meningite Tubercolare," *Arch. Per le Scien. Med.*, Torino, 7th ed., 1 pl. (1883): 59–70.

11. Ludvig Hektoen, "The Vascular Changes of Tuberculous Meningitis, Especially with Tuberculous Endarteritis," *Journal of Experimental Medicine* 1, no. 112 (1896).

12. E. P. Amaral, T. L. Kipnis, E. C. Q. de Carvalho, W. D. da Silva, S. C. Leão, et al., "Difference in Virulence of *Mycobacterium avium* Isolates Sharing Indistinguishable DNA Fingerprint Determined in Murine Model of Lung Infection," PLOS ONE 6, no. 6 (June 2011): e21673.

13. U. F. Rowlatt, "The Effect of Prolonged Tuberculous Meningitis on the Brain and Spinal Cord," *Acta Neuropathologica* 3 (1964): 532–46.

14. M. Elleder, "Chemical Characterization of Age Pigments," in R. S. Sohal (ed.), *Age Pigments* (Amsterdam: Elsevier, North Holland Biomedical Press, 1981), 203–41.

15. S. E. Converse, J. D. Mougous, M. D. Leavell, J. A. Leary, C. R. Bertozzi, and J. S. Cox, "MmpL8 Is Required for Sulfolipid-1 Biosynthesis and *Mycobacterium tuberculosis* Virulence," *Proceedings of the National Academy of Sciences* 100 (2003): 6121–6.

16. A. H. Buck, *A Reference Handbook of the Medical Sciences*, vol. VI (L. William Wood & Company, 1889), 295.

17. W. L. Beatty, E. R. Rhoades, H.-J. Ullrich, D. Chatterjee, J. E. Heuser, et al., "Trafficking and Release of Mycobacterial Lipids from Infected Macrophages," *Traffic* 1 (2000): 235–47.

18. E. E. Southard, "Anatomical Findings in Senile Dementia: A Diagnostic Study Bearing Especially on the Group of Cerebral Atrophies," *American Journal of Insanity* 66, no. 4 (April 1910): 701, 706

19. R. Koch, "Die Atiologie der Tuberkulose," *Berliner Klinische Wochenschrift*, no. I5 (April I0, 1882): 221–230, 227.

CHAPTER 9

Cornell University Department of Immunology. New York City, 1937

Although thoughts that tubercular elements could cause brain plaque and tangles weren't new, they would eventually gain support experimentally.

Jules T. Freund (1890–1960) was a Hungarian-born American immunologist. According to *The Journal of Immunology*, Jules, whose real name was Julius, studied at Budapest's Royal Hungarian University. After receiving his MD degree at the age of twenty-three, he served as a medical intern in the Austrian army (1913–14).

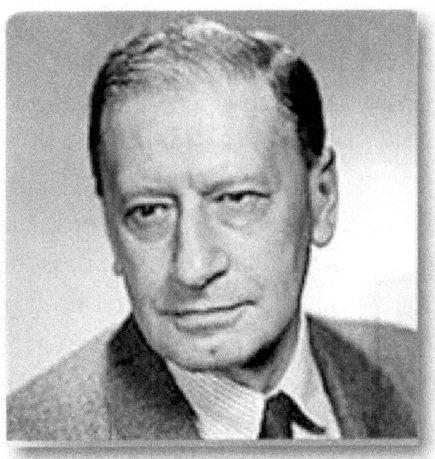

Figure 32. Dr. Jules Freund.

Freund[1] came to the United States on a Harvard fellowship in the Antitoxin and Vaccine Lab in Boston. By 1938, he became Assistant Director of the Department of Health in New York City, eventually working his way up to become the first chief of the Laboratory of Immunology at the National Institute of Allergy and Infectious Diseases (NIAID) in Bethesda, Maryland.

Freund is most remembered for his work on adjuvant techniques for immunization. But to be sure, the ideas and materials he used had been well defined by previous investigators. The word "adjuvant" is from the Latin *adjuvare*—to help. Adjuvants are often included in vaccines, supposedly to enhance the vaccine recipient's "immune response" in an attempt to heighten the vaccine's level of effectiveness. Hopefully adding such an "adjuvant" to a shot would reduce the amount of active foreign material that has to go into the vaccine and thus into the patient.

Freund might have been looking for improved vaccine techniques, but what he developed would be used subsequently experimentally, at least in animals, to induce aspects of a variety of diseases, including neurodegenerative disease — similar to Alzheimer's.

At least initially, Julius Freund's adjuvant included marinating apparently "killed" species of one of the most deadly infectious pathogens in the world, the tubercle bacilli, in oily vehicles. He knew, through the work of previous researchers, that such oily vehicles potentiated the activity of TB. Freund's initial concoction eventually became known as "Complete Freund's Adjuvant" (CFA), with its "killed" TB. Billiau and Matthys, after a thorough review of the literature, stated, "Clearly, the host response to an injection of Complete Freund's Adjuvant (CFA) should be seen as resembling one coping with a slowly fading primary infection with living mycobacteria"[2]—specifically *Mycobacteria tuberculosis.* Billiau and Matthys's caution is well taken. "Heat-killed" tuberculosis and its related mycobacteria, either in vaccination or even as a tuberculin skin test, have dormant, practically indestructible cell-wall-deficient forms that can revert back to virulent TB bacilli—"killed" by neither heat nor sterilization.[3,4,5]

Yet it was just this introduction of tubercular CFA in the late 1940s that quickly became and remains the gold standard for invoking experimental "autoimmune" disease in animals—including the induction of a brain-inflaming, plaque-producing, Experimental Autoimmune Encephalopathy [EAE]. All it took was a single injection of what Freund eventually settled on as brain material mixed with killed tuberculosis in an oily vehicle.

Freund would also go on to develop an "Incomplete" adjuvant without TB in it, subsequently called "Incomplete Freund's Adjuvant" (IFA). But this paled when compared to the "immune response" created by Freund's with TB. The way Freund's Complete Adjuvant works still is not clearly understood; immunologists continue to use it experimentally to create disease in animals, complete with its tubercular components. This lack of understanding is likewise true for Freund's Incomplete Adjuvant without the TB, used again without really knowing or caring how it supposedly "bolsters the immune system" or the exact profile of its side effects. For reasons such as this, Janeway and others have called adjuvants such as Freund's "the immunologist's dirty little secret." As testimony to this, we read paper after paper on Medline involving the obligatory use of tubercular elements to create serious experimental "autoimmune" disease such as EAE—papers in which the use of "dead" tubercular elements are hidden in the Materials and Methods section, only to be seemingly selectively forgotten about in fashioning a concluding discussion.

In the meantime, what currently remains the theory behind how Freund's Complete Adjuvant is thought to work, and how it really works, do not always match. For example, many assume that when the "active" ingredient, such as injected neural material, is introduced into Complete Freund's Adjuvant with TB (CFA) that such CFA adjuvant works merely by increasing such neural or brain material's effective antigenic delivery. This supposedly sets off a complex set of signals to the immune system that alter white-blood-cell proliferation and differentiation. Yet in guinea pigs and mice, the tubercular elements in CFA are mandatory for EAE, and just brain or nervous tissue alone will usually not work.[11]

Thus, it is Freund's Complete Adjuvant, complete with elements of TB, that is needed in experimental models of "autoimmune" diseases, including EAE, an animal model of brain inflammation with a propensity for instigating plaque in the brain, including Alzheimer's neuritic amyloid plaque and tangles.[21]

In addition, several studies have indicated, very conceivably, an association between M. tuberculosis infection and development of "autoimmune" disease itself. [7–10]

———————————

Actually, the idea of injecting tuberculosis into a fatty vehicle such as paraffin oil—Freund's original technique—was first used decades before by Rabinovitch in Koch's laboratory. Rabinovitch had stumbled across the fact that the simple addition of butter into a relatively tame strain of a tubercular-like mycobacterial injection caused a skin reaction almost identical to the most deadly strains of tuberculosis. However, Grasberger soon reported that paraffin oil was far more effective than butter in potentiating injections with such nonpathogenic strains.

Similarly, Dienes and Schoenheit (1926), in an almost forgotten paper,[12] suggested that perhaps an area resembling a tuberculous focus could be created if protein solutions as a vaccine's active ingredient were incorporated with a suspension of paraffin oil into which dead tubercle bacilli had been suspended. By 1935, the Frenchman Coulaud,[13] and four years later Saenz,[16] did just that, following up on Dienes's lead. Certainly neither Dienes nor Coulaud's work escaped Julius Freund, who's Complete Freund's Adjuvant was based upon.

Yet for the time being, Freund, now at Cornell in New York, was running a study with Eugene Opie that concluded that heat-killed human TB could be substituted for Calmette's classic dilute cow tuberculosis vaccination (BCG) against TB. Despite their claimed positive results, Freund and Opie's use of heat-killed tuberculosis for a vaccination caught on no more than Koch's earlier proposal to use heat-killed Old Tuberculin as a vaccine. Yet in that paper, Freund also mentioned—just two years after Coulaud's work— that killed tubercle bacillus injected in combination with a variety of vaccination agents "increase their immunizing activity."[1]

It was only in 1942 that Freund and McDermott[15] used a similar water-in-oil emulsion containing killed *Mycobacteria tuberculosis* that others had used previously in animal experiments. But somehow it was Freund's combination that took the credit, becoming popularly known as Complete Freund's Adjuvant

By 1951, Freund[16] was examining the effect of emulsifying an aqueous solution of the antigen ovalbumin (the main protein found in egg whites) in a paraffin oil containing killed tubercle bacilli with the aid of a surfactant. Oil and water didn't mix. But with a surfactant, one could bring the ingredients involved into suspension. With development, this resulted in Complete Freund's Adjuvant (CFA), a water-in-oil emulsion of mineral oil, mannide monooleate (a surfactant to hold the water-in-oil emulsion together), and heat-killed *Mycobacterium tuberculosis* organisms or components of these organisms. In creating Freund's Complete Adjuvant, Freund had developed a potent adjuvant that stimulated both humoral and cell-mediated immunity. However, he also had on his hands an "immune booster" with supposedly dead tuberculosis, whose toxicity limited its use to laboratory animals. The mineral oil in it could not be metabolized, and the TB, at the very least elicited, in short order, a severe granulomatous reaction.

Although CFA-induced arthritis has been reported in small and large animals,[17-19] the severity of the lesion varied and could be very debilitating, especially in larger animals. Lewis rats injected with heat-killed mycobacterial cells suspended in mineral oil develop polyarthritis, resulting in the term "adjuvant arthritis."[20] By the same token, Julius Freund's CFA, when injected into mice, showed widespread ß-amyloid plaque in the cerebral cortex and hippocampus—the part of the brain that is involved in memory—and within just four months of their being injected.[21]

NOTES

1. Jules Freund, 1890–1960. *The Journal of Immunology* 90, no. 3 (March 1, 1963): NP-33.

2. A. Billiau and P. Matthys, "Modes of Action of Freund's Adjuvants in Experimental Models of Autoimmune Diseases," *Journal of Leukocyte Biology* 70 (December 2001): 851.

3. P. Zwadyk, J. A. Down, N. Myers, et al., "Rendering of Mycobacteria Safe for Molecular Diagnostic Studies and Development of a Lysis Method for Strand Displacement Amplification and PCR," *Journal of Clinical Microbiology* 32 (1994): 2140–6.

4. P. Bemer-Melchior and H. B. Drugeon, "Inactivation of Mycobacterium Tuberculosis for DNA Typing Analysis," *Journal of Clinical Microbiology* 37 (1999): 2350–1.

5. A. P. Lysenko, V. V. Vlasenko, L. Broxmeyer, A. P. Lemish, T. P. Novik, et al., "The Tuberculin Skin Test: How Safe Is Safe?—The Tuberculins Contain Unknown Forms Capable of Reverting to Cell-Wall-Deficient Mycobacteria," *Clinical and Experimental Medical Sciences* 2, no. 2 (2014): 55–73, HIKARI Ltd., www.m-hikari.com, http://dx.doi.org/10.12988/cems.2014.445.

6. C. A. Janeway, Jr., "Approaching the Asymptote? Evolution and Revolution in Immunology," *Cold Spring Harbor Symposia on Quantitative Biology* 54 (1989): 1–13.

7. Y. Shoenfeld and I. Cohen, "Infection and Autoimmunity," in *The Antigens*, vol. VII, edited by M. Sela 88 (1989): 307 Academic Press, New York.

8. J. Holoshitz, Y. Naparstek, A. Ben Nun, and I. R. Cohen, "Lines of T Lymphocytes Induce or Vaccinate against Autoimmune Arthritis," *Science* 219 (1983), 56.

9. H. Teplizki, D. Buskila, S. Argov, D. Isenberg, A. R. M. Coates, S. S. Sukenik, J. Horowitz, and Y. Shoenfeld. "Low Serum Antimycobacterial Glycolipid Antibody Titers in the Sera of Patients with Systemic Lupus Erythematosus Associated with Central Nervous System Involvement," *Journal of Rheumatology* 14 (1987b): 507.

10. D. Buskila, M. Abu-Shakra, H. Amital-Teplizki, A. R. Coates, M. Krupp, *et al.*, "Serum Monoclonal Antibodies Derived from Patients with Multiple Myeloma React with Mycobacterial Phosphoinositides and Nuclear Antigens," *Clinical & Experimental Immunology* 76, no. 3 (1989): 378–83.

11. R. G. White, "Role of Adjuvants in the Production of Delayed Hypersensitivity," *British Medical Bulletin* 23 (1967 Jan) 1: 39–45.

12. L. Dienes and E.W. Schoenheit. "A note on the resistance of specific properties of the tubercle bacillus to sodium hydroxide and hydrochloric acid. With remarks on the relation between antigenic effect in complement fixation and the tuberculin effect." *American Review of Tuberculosis* Vol. 12 (1925 Sept).

13. E. Coulaud, E. (1935) *C. R. Soc. Biol.* 119 (1935): 368–71.

14. E. L. Opie and J. Freund, "An Experimental Study of Protective Inoculation with Heat-Killed Tubercle Bacilli," *Journal of Experimental Medicine* 66, no. 6 (November 30, 1937): 761–88.

15. J. Freund and K. McDermott, K, "But in Reality, Freund's Complete Adjuvant Was Really Coulaud's Complete Adjuvant," *Proceedings of the Society for Experimental Biology and Medicine* 49 (1942): 548–51.

16. J. Freund, "The Effect of Paraffin Oil and Mycobacteria on Antibody Forma tion and Sensitization: A Review," *American Journal of Clinical Pathology* 21 (1951): 645–56.

17. C. M. Pearson, "Development of Arthritis, Periarthritis, and Periostitis in Rats Given Adjuvant," *Proceedings of the Society for Experimental Biology and Medicine* 91 (1956): 95–101.

18. C. M. Pearson and F. D. Wood, "Studies of Polyarthritis and Other Lesions Induced in Rats by Injection of Mycobacterial Adjuvant—I. General Clinical and Pathologic Characteristics and Some Modifying Factors," *Arthritis & Rheumatology* 2 (1959): 440–459; Public Health Service (PHS), 1986.

19. B. H. Waksman, C. M. Pearson, and J. T. Sharp, "Studies of Arthritis and Other Lesions Induced in Rats by Injection of Mycobacterial Adjuvants—II. Evidence That the Disease Is a Disseminated Immunologic Response to Exogenous Antigens," *Journal of Immunology* 85 (1960): 403–17.

20. S. M. Park, J. H. Shin, G. J. Moon, S. I. Cho, Y. B. Lee, et al., "Effects of Collagen-Induced Rheumatoid Arthritis on Amyloidosis and Microvascular Pathology in APP/PS1 Mice," *BMC Neuroscience* 12 (2011): 106.

21. A. Schneider, G. W. Arau'jo, K. Trajkovic, M. M. Herrmann, D. Merkler, E. Mandelkow, R. Weissert, and M. Simons, "Hyperphosphorylation and Aggregation of Tau in Experimental Autoimmune Encephalomyelitis," *The Journal of Biological Chemistry* 279, no. 53 (December 31, 2004): 55833–9.

CHAPTER 10

The Guam Memorial Hospital, US Territory of Guam, 1965

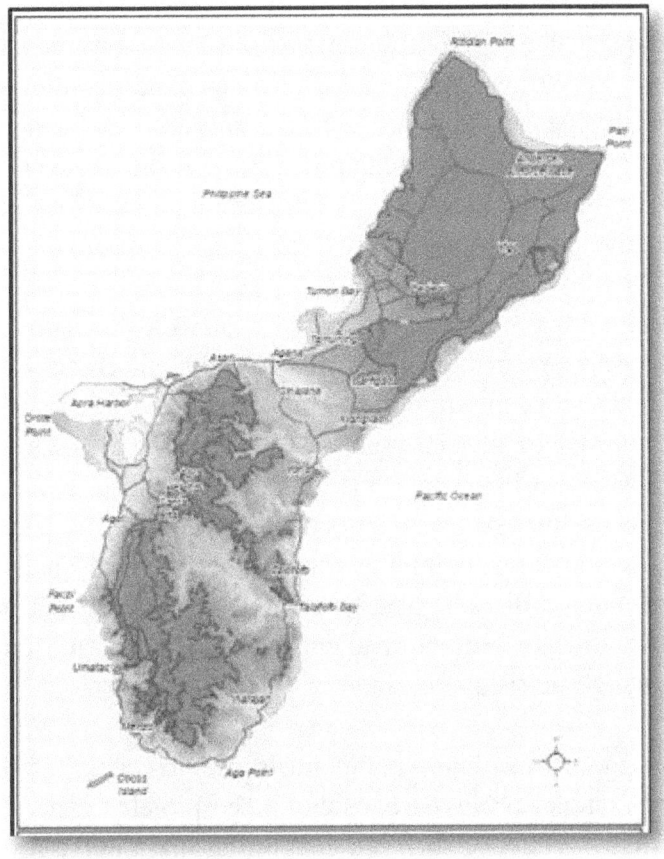

Figure 33. US Territory of Guam.

Dr. Alzheimer's disease was not the only one showing cerebral neurofibrillary tangles. Such tangles were also seen in postencephalitic parkinsonism, other diseases of postencephalitis, progressive supranuclear palsy, amyotrophic lateral sclerosis (also known as ALS or Lou Gehrig's disease), neurotuberculosis, and the ALS–Parkinson's–dementia complex of Guam, a disease first recorded on Guam in 1904.

Guam is located in the southernmost Marianas, a tropical island chain in the Western Pacific region, fifteen hundred miles east of the Philippines and eighteen hundred miles south of Japan. It is part of an underwater mountain range and is the largest of more than two thousand islands between Hawaii and the Philippines. The native people of Guam are known as "Chamorros."

Although it had been present for more than 150 years on Guam, it was only since the middle of the twentieth century that a remarkable concentration of cases of the neurodegenerative disease referred to officially as the ALS–Parkinson's–Dementia complex (ALS/PDC) of Guam was recognized among the Chamorros. Intense investigations have since failed to determine its cause, but at one point it affected 10 percent of the natives on Guam. Such a disease, had it occurred in the America of that day, would have been equivalent to twenty-seven million victims, a nightmarish scenario.

Furthermore, the major components of Alzheimer's neurofibrillary tangles are hyperphosphorylated proteins called "tau." Eventually, evidence surfaced suggesting that the tau found in the mysterious neurodegenerative disease on Guam was similar to that observed in Alzheimer's.[1]

When in the early eighteenth century Spain went after Magellan's stake in earnest, war broke out on the island of Guam. But it was not through combat that the Chamorro population was decimated from a total of 70,000 to 1,634 by the year 1700.[2] Without doubt, the main cause of the devestation of the Chamorro population on Guam were epidemics such as smallpox and TB brought in by the Spaniards.[3] Guam was not alone, and it is clear that the populations of not only the Pacific Islands but the New World itself had not developed the necessary antibodies to confront Old World illness. The American Indians were also no strangers to killer epidemics imported from Europe, such as when their reservations were converted into tubercular infernos of death, reaching a mortality by 1913 ten times higher than anything that Europe had seen in the worst of its nineteenth-century epidemics—a tubercular mortality rate that reached the highest rate anywhere at any time.[4]

By the late eighteenth century, Filipino immigration to Guam had created a situation in which approximately one in five Chamorros were direct descendents of Filipino–Chamorro unions[5]—a small token of what was to follow. World War II's conclusion saw a Filipino influx that reached ten thousand by 1970. Soon it was discovered that after a mean lapse of decades, Filipinos were also contracting the mysterious PD–Dementia on Guam. Garruto's 1981 question[6] was "Were people importing the disease from the Philippines?" It had already been concluded that the overwhelming majority of these neurodegenerative diseases originally occurred in the setting of an upper respiratory tract infection, a headache, and frequently a prolonged Fever of Unknown Origin (FUO)[7]—long known to be characteristic of a tubercular involvement, so prevalent in the Philippines to begin with.

Since America's original occupation of Guam, one particular health concern surfaced at the Navy Department:

> Naval Station, Guam, L.I.—Reports from the island of Guam show progressive, steady improvement in health conditions since the American occcupation. During the year 1916 there were no cases of pneumonia or pleurisy; no typhoid fever; no acute exanthemata. The birth rate is on the increase, and there is a slight reduction in the mortality figures in spite of tuberculosis, which threatens to become a serious factor. It is with regret that we notice the increasing prevalence of this disease on Guam.[8]

Guam was heavily populated with both Japanese and American military forces during World War II. The immediate post-World War II period was one of reconstruction and redevelopment Pacificwide, and these activities were particularly apparent on Guam. Commercial air traffic was reestablished, and there was a steady influx of Filipino laborers from Luzon.

World War II was over, yet this deadly neurological disease plagued the small island of Guam. The natives called it "lytico-bodig"—"lytico" from the Spanish word *paralytico*, which means weakness. The "bodig" referred to signs of Parkinson's dementia. But patients could have features of Lou Gehrig's Disease (ALS), Parkinson's, and Alzheimer's diseases—a melding of symptoms causing paralysis, sluggishness, and forgetfulness. Endemic to the native population of Chamorros, the ALS portion of the syndrome alone was at one point fifty to one hundred times more prevalent on Guam than anywhere else in the world. After ruling out a genetic cause, scientists began the hunt for an environmental trigger. A staple of the local cuisine raised suspicion. Then there was a focus on abnormal minerals and metals in the soil. The water and food of Guam were scrutinized. So too came the inevitable search for a "virus."

Elizan mentions that in 1962, Russian virus hunter Zilber (actual spelling Zil'ber) and his virologist associates reported in the Russian virology journal *Voprosy Virusologii* on the possibe viral etiology of amyotrophic lateral sclerosis. One year later, in 1963, Zilber et al. reappeared[10] with the same article, this time in English and without the words "Possible Viral Etiology" in their title, but with much the same intent of suggesting that a virus was responsible. Zilber was aware of the Guam studies, which seemed divided at the time as to whether the Amyotrophic Lateral Sclerosis–Parkinson's dementia complex on Guam was genetic or "toxinfectious." To Zilber's group, "toxinfectious" meant it was probably, but not certainly, viral—and they actually suceeded in transferring the disease's infectious agent from spinal and medulla homogenates of patients who had died from ALS to monkeys. But this was only after a latent period of what Zilber estimated in his conclusion to be from one to five years, or more (Zilber, 1963). Also in his conclusion, Zilber modified his insistance on the infectious agent being a virus by using the more vague term "virus-like." However, the methods used by Zilber and his group toward ruling out a bacterial or particularly a viral-like, cell-wall-deficient, mycobacterial cause seem unclear. In fact, no tubercular mycobacterial tests were as much as mentioned in the paper. And a bacterial cause was dismissed with just as much casualness. Zilber wrote the following:

All bacteriological tests of the medullary [and spinal] material remained fruitless. The material from human beings and from passages in monkeys was administered with antibiotics. Thus the idea that the causative agent is bacterial in nature may be excluded, and we may assert that a viral agent is concerned.[10]

But in reality, Zilber excluded nothing, only introducing the antibiotics penicillin and streptomycin into the infected brain and spinal cord material just before placing it into the brains of monkeys through a skull trephine hole. This combination of antibiotics certainly did not in any way "exclude" a bacterial or a mycobacterial infection. In the face of the innate resistance of a nerve-seeking strain of mycobacterial infection, simply administering penicillin and streptomycin would have merely delayed the microbe's growth and certainly not killed it. Furthermore, other labs could not reproduce Zilber's viral hypothesis—nor were any known viral antibodies being picked up. Yet the fact remained that Zilber had established that some infectious agent was causing the crippling disease on Guam, and one seasoned investigator surmised that it was probably caused by some infectious encephalitis.

This much we know. By July 1946, one-half of the people in Guam hospitals were suffering from tuberculosis.[11] And by 1954, Mulder and Kurland admitted that TB was a leading cause of death on Guam and that TB meningitis was frequently seen in its hospitals.[7] At least a comparable situation existed in the Philippines, where one of the highest rates of tubercular incidence and prevalence in the world existed.

Long the principal killer on Guam, from 1905 to 1970, deaths from TB exceeded the number of deaths from all epidemics occurring on the Island. Even as late as 1952, TB was the greatest single killer on the island. To be certain, tuberculosis was also prevelent in Japan, which toward the end of the war sent nineteen thousand troops into Guam in an effort to repel the final American counterinvasion. To further complicate matters, Silva-Krott et al. (1998) eventually determined that *M. avium* or fowl tuberculosis also exists on Guam in certain bird species,[12] and there were more than enough "bird biting" mosquito vectors available to transmit and translate this into human disease. The mosquito *Culex quinquefasciatus* is widespread on Guam,[13] and like the *Aedes aegypti* mosquito, it was known on Guam since the early 1900s.[14] But it was *Culex quinquefasciatus*, unlike the *Aedes aegypti*, that had the capacity to bite both birds and humans.

Tuberculosis on Guam was brought under control within the same window of time in which the mysterious ALS–PDC on Guam also steeply declined, between 1950 and 1960 — after which both TB and the shadowy neurodegenerative disease on Guam both declined.[15] It seemed that no one born after 1951 developed or was at risk of developing the ALS-PDC on Guam. Clearly, its existence as an epidemic ended on Guam because whatever its cause or mode of transmission was had also ended. But exactly what had changed and led to this?

Oddly enough, then, just before this abrupt decline in incidence of Guam's mysterious nervous disorder, a massive mosquito-control program with the ultra-effective DDT insecticide was instituted on the island in the 1940s. Insect-related diseases, huge on Guam before the use of massive amounts of DDT by air starting in August 1944, sunk dramatically. This aerial DDT campagin singlehandledly all but wiped out an entire mosquito species—the dangerous *Aedes aegypti*—to the point that only a single specimen of the *A. Aegypti* mosquito was recovered on Guam in a 1950 survey. It also decimated Culex species of mosquitoes. *Aedes aegypti* would not even begin to recover again until the 1970s.[16]

It is strange, then, that it went widely unnoticed that mosquitoes such as *Aedes aegypti* and the species Culex can also transmit tubercular-like mycobacterial disease.[17–20]

The fact that tuberculosis and the other mycobacteria can be transmitted through mosquito vectors is no longer an uncertainty, yet because the pathogen changes forms while inside the mosquito, it was still being widly rejected as transmissible. Yet is was just such slow-growing cell-wall-deficient mycobacteria, originating from a mosquito, that could explain exactly how an infection could exist, give no symptoms when the infection begins, and silently advance with a very long latency that might take decades before becoming evident.

Bloodsucking insects such as mosquitoes can be significant vectors for many infectious diseases, and mycobacteria such as *Mycobacterium tuberculosis* are no exception. Golyshevskaya[21] described how, during blood suction after the sting of an *Aedes aegypti* mosquito, he saw classic rod-shapped mycobacterial bacilli change into small, ultrafine, viral-like coccoid forms that were spherical in shape. Such tubercular/mycobacterial forms have a dense cellular membrane often mistaken for the capsid of a virus. Although they can revert back to the classical tubercullar bacilli at any time, their main usefulness inside the propagating mosquito was both the resiliance of such tiny cell-wall-deficient coccoid forms while in the mosquito, and, as a side benefit, they also made mycobacterial transmission easier through the mosqito while sucking blood.

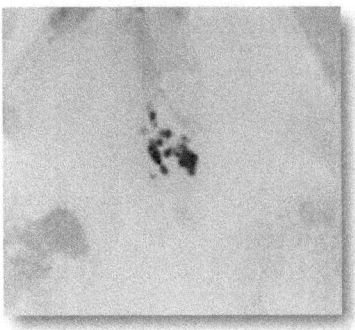

Figure 34. Small darkly stained, circular-shaped, cell-wall-deficient mycobacterial forms.

With the DDT decimation of *Aedes aegypti* and *Culex quinque-fasciatus*, the two main avenues of man-to-mosquito-to-man and bird-to-mosquito-to-man mycobacterial intrusion had been ripped from the ongoing mosquito offensive on Guam. In addition, the brown tree snake (*Boiga irregularis*), introduced fortuitously at the end of World War II, was wreaking havoc on Guam's Micronesian Kingfisher and the Guam rail populations—the two main potential avian repositories for possible bird-to-mosquito-to-human fowl tuberculosis. Although kingfishers were collected and observed in southern Guam in 1945, their numbers decreased sharply over the next two decades. Because these brown tree-snake reptiles had no natural predators on Guam, their numbers grew, and they spread across the island quickly. Within three decades, therefore, they hunted Micronesian kingfishers and eight other bird species to the brink of extinction.

So if the the ALS–Parkinson's–dementia complex of Guam to this day remains a mystery, so too was the complete lack of scientific pursuit in a mycobacterial direction, mosquito-borne or not, to explain what really had happened on Guam.

NOTES

1. V. Buee-Scherrer, L. Buee, P. R. Hof, B. Leveugle, C. Gilles, et al., "Neurofibrillary Degeneration in Amyotrophic Lateral Sclerosis/Parkinsonism-Dementia Complex of Guam: Immunochemical Characterization of Tau Proteins," *American Journal of Pathology* 146, no. 4 (April 1995): 924–32.

2. S. Schoeder, "Admiral Seaton Schoeder's Tour of Duty, *Guam Recorder* 3 (1926): 36.

3. F. X. Hezel, "From Conversion to Conquest: The Early Spanish Mission in the Marianas," Journal of Pacific History 17, no. 3 (1982): 115–37.

4. J. B. McDougall, *Tuberculosis: A Global Study in Social Pathology* (Edinburgh: E&S Livingstone Ltd., 1950).

5. R. M. Garruto, "Amyotrophic Lateral Sclerosis and Parkinson–Dementia among Filipino Migrants to Guam," *Annals of Neurology* 10 (1981): 341–50.

6. S. Lessell "Seizure in a Guamanian Village," *Archives of Neurology* 7 (1962): 37–44.

7. D. W. Mulder and L. T. Kurland, "Neurologic Diseases on Island of Guam," *US Armed Forces Medical Journal* 5 (1954): 1724–39.

8. *Annual Reports of the Navy Department for the Fiscal Year 1917* (Washington: Government Printing Office, 1918), 769.

9. L. A. Zilber, et al., "Possible Viral Etiology of Amyotrophic Lateral Sclerosis," *Voprosy Virusologii* 5 (October 1962): 520–8.

10. L. A. Zilber, Z. L. Bajdakova, A. N. Gardasjan, N. V. Konovalov, T. L. Bunina, et al., "Study of the Etiology of Amyotrophic Lateral Sclerosis," *Bulletin of the World Health Organization Journal* 29 (1963): 449–56.

11. H. Jacobziner, "Tuberculosis Program on Guam including an All-Island Tuberculin Patch Test Study," *Naval Medical Bulletin* 48, no. 5 (September–October 1948): 700–21.
12. I. M. Silva-Krott, K. Brock, and R. E. Junge. "Determination of the Presence of *Mycobacterium avium* on Guam as Precursor to Reintroduction of Indigenous Bird Species, *Pacific Conservation Biology* 4 (1998): 227–31.
13. L. M. Rueda, J. E. Pecor, W. K. Reeves, S. P. Wolf, P. V. Nunn, R. Y. Rabago, T. L. Gutierrez, and M. Debboun, "Mosquitoes of Guam and the Northern Marianas: Distribution, Checklists, and Notes on Mosquito-Borne Pathogens," *The Army Medical Department Journal* (July–September 2011): 17–28.
14. J. F. Leys, "Report on the United States Naval Station, Island of Guam, (1904)," in *Annual) Report of the Surgeon General, US Navy (for 1905)* (1905): 91–6; Bureau of Medicine & Surgery, US Navy Department, Washington, DC.
15. C. C. Plato, R. M. Garruto, D. Galasko, U. K. Craig, M. Plato, et al., "Amyotrophic Lateral Sclerosis and Parkinsonism-Dementia Complex of Guam: Changing Incidence Rates during the Past Sixty Years," *American Journal of Epidemiology* 157, no. 2 (2003): 149–157.
16. W. R. Nowell, "Comparative Mosquito Collection Data from the Southern Mariana Islands (Diptera: Culicidae)," *Proceedings of the California Mosquito and Vector Control Association* 48 (1980): 112–6.
17. R. Banerjee, B. D. Banerjee, S. Chaudhury, and A. K. Hati AK, "Transmission of Viable *Mycobacterium leprae* by *Aedes aegypti* from Lepromatous Leprosy Patients to the Skin of Mice through Intermittent Feeding," *Tropical and Geographical Medicine* 42 (1991): 97–9.

18. E. Narayanan, K. S. Manja, W. F. Kirchheimer, and M. Balasubrahmanyan, "Occurance of *Mycobacterium leprae* in Arthropods," *Leprosy Review* 43 (1972): 194–8.
19. E. Narayanan, Sreevatsa, W. F. Kirchheimer, and B. M. Bedi, "Transfer of Leprosy Bacilli from Patients to Mouse Footpads by *Aedes aegypti,*" *Leprosy Review* 49 (1977): 181–6.
20. E. Narayanan E, Sreevatsa, A. D. Raj, W. F. Kirchheimer, and B. M. Bedi, "Persistence and Distribution of *Mycobacterium leprae* in *Aedes aegypti* and *Culex fatigans* Experimentally Fed on Leprosy Patients," *Leprosy* 50 (India) (1978): 26–37.
21. V. I. Golyshevskaya, "The Role of Coccoid Ultrafine Forms of Mycobacteria in the Transmission of the Mycobacterial Infection," *Pneumoftiziologia* 40, no. 4 (October–December 1991): 11–13.

CHAPTER 11

Office of Medical Research Director, the State Institute for Geriatrics, Warren, Pennsylvania, 1972

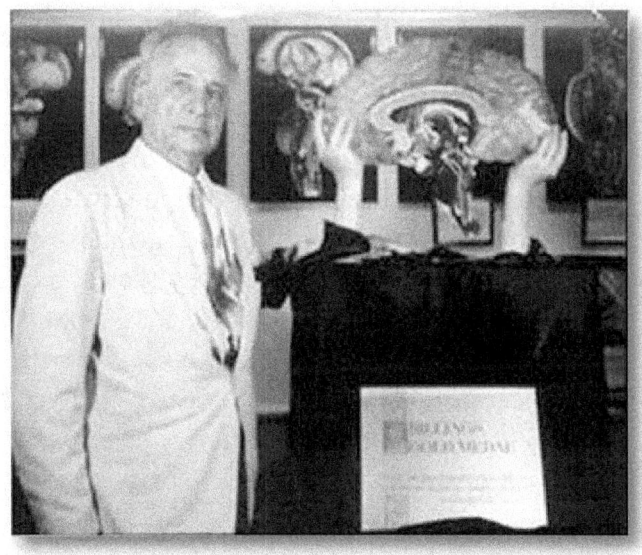

Figure 35. Professor Dr. Med. Philipp Schwartz American Medical Association Award USA, 1960.

As he read Oskar Fischer's turn-of-the-century study in the 1970s, nothing, including Fischer's referencing a tubercle, and the "miliary" tubercular-like distribution of Alzheimer's brain plaque, seemed out of order to Pennsylvania neuropathologist Philip Schwartz. Nor could he find any fault in Southard's Alzheimer's autopsy conclusions at Harvard or Clouston's original research implying Alzheimer and the senile dementias as being a result of old and mostly dormant foci of TB. Rather, Schwartz's findings were comparable. Schwartz made this observation:

> Chronic infections, and particularly tuberculosis, have heretofore been regarded as the most frequent and therefore the most important cause of systemic amyloid degeneration. This fact induced us to look for sequels of pulmonary tuberculosis in around 150 cases of senile and presenile [Alzheimer's] amyloidosis. Postmortem roentgen photography, as well as careful macroscopic and histologic examination of the lungs, disclosed typical calcifications of healed intra-pulmonary or lymphoglandular tuberculous infiltrates in almost every instance of this series, and quite often typical cicatrices of old lymphonodular bronchial lesions. *Doubtless, the great majority of our senile and presenile patients displaying cerebral amyloidosis, suffered from pulmonary tuberculosis sometimes before symptoms of senile deterioration arose.*[1]

Among those first fired from their jobs by the Nazis in 1933 was Hungarian-born Frankfurt pathologist Dr. Philip Schwartz. Schwartz, then a full professor in Frankfurt-am-Main, who ironically worked in the same city where Alzheimer first observed Frau Auguste Deter. Unlike Oskar Fischer, however, Schwartz clearly saw Nazi intentions, sensibly fleeing to Switzerland. There he established the Notgemeinschaft Deutscher Wissenschaftler im

Ausland, the Emergency Assistance Organization for German Scientists, to help Jewish and other persecuted German scholars secure employment in countries prepared to receive them.

Turkey, interested in revamping its science, architecture, music, and medicine, was a prime consideration. Turkey had always been predisposed to German science and culture because of longstanding ties between the two countries. And so it was that Turkey invited Philip Schwartz to Ankara for government-level meetings—leading to the resettlement of himself and twenty-nine other displaced German scientists to Ankara. Later, through the tireless help of Albert Einstein, this number was increased to 180.

Originally a Swiss pathologist, Schwartz, a student of Löeffler, having completed his work in Ankara, moved to the United States to become Director of Research at the Pennsylvania State Institute in Warren. There, through extensive human and animal autopsy-driven studies, Schwartz almost invariably found tubercular foci in Alzheimer's bodies—usually latent. Though seemingly dormant, he knew that such foci could reactivate at any time, leading through either immunologic mechanisms or direct systemic invasion to tissue changes identical to those seen by Fischer and Alzheimer.[1] It is unclear why the elites of American medicine shelved Schwartz's extensive and well-documented neuropathological work on Alzheimer's, other than the fact that it brought up a topic both out of their comfort zone and interest—a wider role for cerebral tuberculosis.

Schwartz marveled not only at how psychiatry had become isolated within the framework of medicine, but moreover, psychiatric complacency with regard to internists' and family physicians' almost-reflexive use of the vague diagnosis "Chronic Brain Syndrome," a term that had fast become the standard medical explanation for the age-related dementias. Also, although psychiatric training ideally considered exploration of mental status as well as bodily conditions that could affect one's mental status, it seemed that in practice it was the mental status of a patient alone that was much more important to the profession. Philip Schwartz thought this left "no real psychiatric incentive to explore tuberculosis or any other direct infectious etiologic cause underlying senile and presenile dementia."[2]

Nor was Schwartz particularly impressed by Kraepelin's attempts at creating a tidy, compartmentalized psychiatric classification system. Rather, in the real world, Schwartz concluded, the same cerebral amyloid pathology that existed in say dementia praecox or schizophrenia with time could morph into Alzheimer's presenile and then senile dementia. Schwartz said this:

> We have shown that Alzheimer's disease and common mental deterioration are associated with cerebral amyloid deposits. Thus, psychiatric conditions, which we consider to be important because of their high incidence are linked to organic cerebral alterations. Practically all psychotic symptoms observed in younger patients suffering from schizophrenia or paranoia are found also in Alzheimer's disease and in common senile dementia.[1, p. 130]

This led him to make this conclusion:

> It seems to us that a thorough and unbiased analysis of basic psychotic symptoms like hallucinations, morbid ideation, asocial behavior and autistic thinking will be useful not only for the characterization of presenile and senile deterioration, but also for a new evaluation of psychiatric conditions in general.[1]

One of the main reasons why Dr. Philip Schwartz could go where few had gone before him was his introduction of a critical method, still used today, whereby the flourochrome dye Thioflavin-S lit up amyloid deposits, both in humans and animals. Using this process, Schwartz proceeded to fashion the textbook *Amyloidosis: Cause and Manifestation of Senile Deterioration*—which stands as a monument to the course that solid basic research on Alzheimer's and the amyloid neurodegenerative disorders could have taken.

Neurosyphilis had diminished to a point of rarity, and Schwartz saw amyloidosis—both "primary" (supposedly noninfectious) and secondary (infectious)—in the brain and elsewhere, mostly as the by-product of underlying infectious tuberculosis, usually dormant. Such infection could then, with time or age, either reactivate itself or be reactivated by a host of traumatic, chemical, biologic, or physical insults. He had autopsied hundreds of cases. In each case, animal or human, he documented plaque in the brain, accompanied by the amyloid degeneration of nerve fibrils as a result of systemic infection.

Schwartz injected *M. tuberculosis* into the peritoneal sac of twenty-two guinea pigs, all of whom died within twenty-eight to ninety-six days.[2] All but four exhibited amyloidosis. Yet only one of his control animals came down with amyloidosis. With his guinea pig experiment, Schwartz supported the findings of Hass, who in a large series of rabbits found that three out of every four animals developed amyloidosis within fifteen days of being infected with bovine tuberculosis. Furthermore, the injection of tuberculin into Haas's animals only hastened the development of amyloidosis.[3]

Dr. George M. Hass became chairman of Chicago Presbyterian's Department of Pathology in January 1946. A native of Iowa, he served as an instructor on the faculty at Harvard for seven years, after which he became assistant professor of pathology at Cornell Medical School for three years. In his multipart amyloid study for the *Archives of Pathology*, Hass and his colleagues made this conclusion:

> In the present investigation, the only infectious disease which served as an apparent cause of amyloidosis was tuberculosis.[3, p.228]

All twenty-one of Hass's human subjects with amyloid disease had chronic pulmonary tuberculosis due to the human tubercle bacillus.

———————————————

Philip Schwartz continued to see theoretical discrepancies all about him.

Supposedly, it was out there that the vast majority of Alzheimer's (AD) cases—more than 95 percent—have no defining genetic factor and were considered sporadic, or late-onset. On the other hand, early-onset or familial AD (FAD) referred to a small subset of patients with a supposed genetic component. However, both familial and sporadic forms displayed the same cellular pathological characteristics: amyloid plaques, composed of Aβ peptides; and neurofibrillary tangles. This suggested that they are one and the same and arose through similar mechanisms. By 1994, Frecker, Pryse-Phillips, and Strong, in the *Canadian Journal of Neurological Science*, said that adult exposure to tuberculosis appeared to be a major risk factor for familial dementia of the Alzheimer-type patients. Necessarily, their study also concluded that such TB exposure might be of further relevance in subgroups of nonfamilial Alzheimer patients as well.[4]

Despite claims otherwise, Schwartz knew that bacteria were powerful inflammatory stimulators and that chronic bacterial amyloidosis was the most common form of human systemic amyloidosis worldwide. He summed things up accordingly: "It seems that no one who lives long enough escapes it."

Schwartz steadfastly stood by Divry when Divry was in a decades-long struggle against the medical authorities that amyloid was in fact instrumental in the age-related dementias. In his book's dedication, Schwartz wrote this:

Based on exact and consistent investigation since 1927, Professor Doctor P. Divry of Liège, Belgium has stated that cortical plaques and neuronal Alzheimer fibrils in senile dementia, as well as in Alzheimer's disease, are manifestations of a cerebral amyloid degeneration. He also has found that amyloid deposits affect cerebral vessels and the ependymal and choroidal epithelium. In spite of the fact that his reports were ignored and the correctness of his observations doubted or denied, Divry has patiently and indefatigably persevered in presenting the truth for more than three decades. I am happy to confirm Divry's discoveries.[1]

And Philip Schwartz, having just discovered amyloid-seeking fluorescent Thioflavin-S, was in an excellent position to do just that:

If our fluorescence microscopic investigations were instrumental in the general acceptance of Divry's [amyloid/Alzheimer's] teachings, it was not only the morphological manifoldness of our results but also the extraordinarily large number of cases of common senile dementia and Alzheimer's disease in which we detected the presence of cerebral and extracerebral amyloid. Our confirmation was based not on a few and perhaps rare cases, but on hundreds of routine autopsies."[1 p. 291]

Yet as late as 1967, just three years later, an editorial in the *Journal of the American Medical Association* concluded that "Amyloid disease will never enjoy more than casual clinical importance."[1, p. vii]

Schwartz chaffed at *JAMA*'s inference:

"Our investigations have disclosed amyloidosis to be one of the most frequent diseases of the human species, and *cerebral amyloidosis*, because of its enormous incidence in the aged, to be the most important condition in neuropathology." And Since tuberculosis could still be considered the most frequent infection which produced amyloid deposits and Schwartz had repeatedly documented "Extinct or still active sequels of pulmonary tuberculosis present in almost every case of senile deterioration investigated postmortem", [p 363] his conclusion was inevitably that there was an indelible linkage between Alzheimer's and systemic tuberculosis.

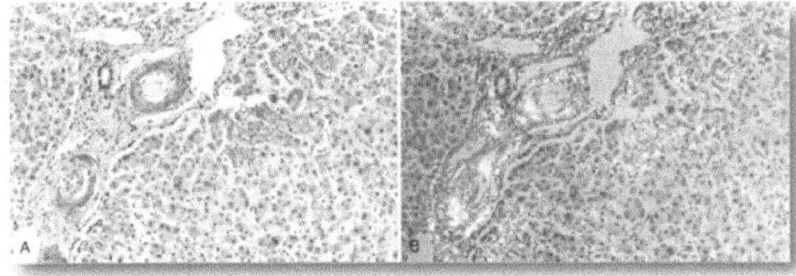

Figure 36. Amyloidosis. Slide A shows section of the liver stained with Congo red revealing deposits of amyloid in the walls of blood vessels and along sinusoids. In slide B, note the birefringence of the deposits when observed by polarizing microscope.

Nor did evolving "classifications" of amyloid, which began in the early 1930s, sidetrack him. Such classifications began with Lubarsch in 1929. But Lubarsch had been woefully wrong in his amyloid assessments in the past. In this classification, amyloid from a chronic disease such as tuberculosis was now being called "secondary" or infectious amyloidosis. This automatically made the whole diagnosis of "primary (noninfectious) amyloidosis" basically one of exclusion and simply meant not that no infection was present but that no infection could be detected. Schwartz's contention was that in all cases, not enough diagnostic and complete autopsy results were performed in these so-called "primary" cases of amyloidosis to attempt to locate their underlying infectious nature. Schwartz wrote this:

> We feel that a systemic inquiry may have revealed healed or still active tuberculous pulmonary processes in many cases recorded as "primary" [noninfectious] or "atypical" amyloidosis.

The diagnosis and finding the real cause for Alzheimer's should have been child's play, neuropathologist Schwartz thought, were it not for the fact that its earlier investigators—perhaps with the exception of Southard and Fischer—were more interested in documenting pathology than finding out what was behind that pathology. And this was only compounded by later researchers whose classifications and speculations regarding amyloid served more, in Schwartz's eyes as obstacles, than to really ascertain what was really behind the amyloid of Alzheimer's.

Schwartz wasn't the only one who remained unimpressed by the specious, ever-changing classifications of amyloidosis that had emerged. According to Jones,[5] the questionable classification of amyloidosis into "primary" [no infectious cause able to be seen] as opposed to traditional and now so-called "secondary" [infectious cause able to be seen] was introduced by Hobart

A. Reimann[6] in 1935. But in that same year, Reimann was still documenting a case of tuberculosis that had caused amyloidosis, as well as citing similar tubercular cause by other authors.[7] To Philip Schwartz, the reason for the flaws in Reimann's classification of amyloid differentiation were more than obvious because often the underlying disease was not found. Thus, Reimann's "noninfectious [primary] causes" have been challenged and rechallenged in the literature as really being of infectious origin. Jones cited that 50 percent of forty cases of infectious amyloidosis reported from Scotland where of tuberculous origin, with no telling what percentage more was from dormant or nondetected cell-wall-deficient forms of the microbe. Jones found subsequent attempts at classification just as unreliable. Yet Jones said that, at the end of the day all amyloid fibrils appeared to have a "beta-pleated sheet" configuration, their unifying factor.

The pitfalls of such a "primary" noninfectious amyloidosis were further documented by Chee, Gertz et al., among others.[8] Chee warned that physicians needed to be aware of clinical scenarios that can mimic but not be "primary" noninfectious amyloidosis "to avoid misdiagnosis and harm to the patient." Such classification, Schwartz agreed, seemed designed to tell us that "primary" amyloid in humans differed from "secondary" amyloidosis, leading one to the conclusion that essentially infection could not, in general, cause a disease like Alzheimer's.

But a closer look at such classification "experts" showed inconsistencies in their own work. For example, Reimann's 1935 watershed publication, sadly lacking, cites a single case of a recent converter to positive tuberculin with a fever of unknown origin and hilar adenopathy. Yet he did no acid-fast stains or any other measures to rule out tuberculosis and somehow came around to calling the case "primary" amyloidosis. In Reimann's opinion, what cinched such a noninfectious origin for amyloid in that case was the finding of "amyloid tongue." This, claimed Reimann, led to the "clinical recognition of the case here reported." Yet since, "amyloid tongue has been found to also occur from infectious cause."[9] Were such classification flaws and loopholes uncommon, they might have been considered anecdotal, but the numbers involved were anything but anecdotal, and Philip Schwartz knew this. Schwartz realized that such classifications regarding the cause of amyloid was no small debate. A misdiagnosis could mean ultimate death.

In the meantime, amyloidosis associated with tuberculosis has long been known to undergo remission and disappear when the chronic tubercular infection has been eliminated.[10]

NOTES

1. P. Schwartz, *Amyloidosis—Cause and Manifestation of Senile Deterioration* (Springfield, Illinois: Charles C Thomas, 1970), 363.
2. P. Schwartz, "Amyloid Degeneration and Tuberculosis in the Aged," *Gerontologia* 18, nos. 5–6 (1972): 321–62.
3. G. M. Hass, and R. Huntington, "Amyloid 111: The Properties of Amyloid Deposits Occurring in Several Species under Diverse Conditions," *Archives of Pathology*35 (1943): 226–41.
4. M. F. Frecker, W. E. M. Pryse-Phillips, and H. R. Strong, "Immunological Associations in Familial and Nonfamilial Alzheimer Patients and Their Families," *Canadian Journal of Neurological Sciences* 21 (1994): 1112–9.
5. N. F. Jones, "Renal Amyloidosis," *Journal of Clinical Pathology* 34 (1981): 1228–32.
6. H. A. Reimann, R. F. Koucky, and C. M. Eklund, "Primary Amyloidosis Limited to Tissue of Mesodermal Origin," American Journal of Pathology 11 (November 1935): 977–88.
7. H. A. Reimann, "Recovery from Amyloidosis," *Journal of the American Medical Association* 104 (1935): 1070–1.
8. C. E. Chee, M. Q. Lacy, D. Ahmet, S. R. Zeidenrust, and M. A. Gertz, "Pitfalls in the Diagnosis of Primary Amyloidosis," *Clinical Lymphoma, Myeloma, and Leukemia*" 10, no. 3 (2010): 177–80.
9. M. I. Cengiz, H. L. Wang, and L. Yildiz, "Oral Involvement in a Case of AA Amyloidosis: A Case Report," *Journal of Medical Case Reports* 4 (June 30, 2010) 200.
10. H. Waldenström, "On the Formation and Disappearance of Amyloid in Man," *Acta Chirurgica Scandinavica* 63 (1928): 479–530.

CONCLUSION

Throughout Alois Alzheimer's papers, it is both remarkable and frankly inexplicable that despite the available, huge amount of peer studies done on tubercular attack on the brain and the nervous system—degenerative or otherwise—Alzheimer never considered this disease in any of the differential diagnoses found in his many publications. Thus, although neurologist/psychiatrist/pathologist Alois Alzheimer was technically excellent in his neuropathological presentations, his laboratory preparations, and their assessment, he seemed lacking in his differential diagnosis. But, then again, even scientific icons can be mistaken.

By late 1912, Alzheimer, who had been appointed as the Chair of Psychiatry at the University of Breslau, took on the case[1] of a twenty-seven-year-old woman of slow speech and weakness who experienced frequent vomiting. Soon afterward, this patient experienced a noticeable stiffness in her gait, with accompanying weakness and sharp, intermittent, spasmodic pains in her left arm, which had increased in intensity. Alzheimer noted that she was depressed, often crying, which, in turn, sometimes resulted in convulsions. She was first sent to a tuberculosis sanatorium and then released to Dr. Ludwig Mann's private office. From there, and for questionable reasons, she found her way into a psychiatric clinic for a consult with Dr. Alzheimer—although Alzheimer admitted that she seemed completely rational and oriented when she was seen. In December 1911, her father died, and she was understandably shocked by the event. Yet Alzheimer made no attempt to chart the cause of her father's death.

So we have a young person, seriously physically sick, sent for a psychiatric evaluation. This in itself could go a long way in explaining her depression and crying. She was seeking a cure for a physical illness, and that cure seemed unreachable. After treatment in the TB sanatorium, she mentioned that there was temporary improvement, but it did not last long; her disease returned with a vengeance. Alzheimer also charted that when she swallowed, it was often the wrong way, and apparently food got "up her nose," a sign that Alzheimer realized showed possible bulbar involvement. But there was also the possibility of spinal involvement, causing what Alzheimer noted as "painful spastic convulsive states of extremities." The term "bulbar" means of or relating to a bulb, specifically involving the medulla oblongata, often called simply the medulla. The spine sits just below the medulla.

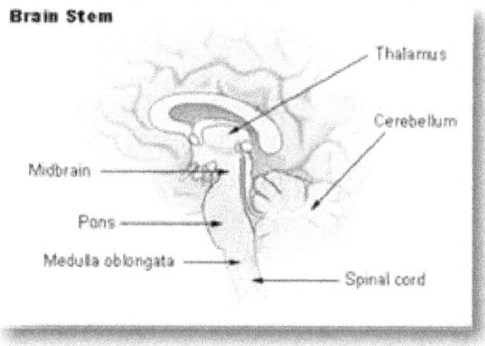

Figure 37. Diagrammatic picture of the midbrain, the medulla (medulla oblongata) and just beneath this, the spinal cord. Symptomwise, the twenty-seven-year-old seemed to be suffering from an attack on or pathology of the medulla and the spine.

As for this patient's frequent vomiting, the medulla houses the chemoreceptor trigger zone (CTZ), which communicates with other structures in the vomiting center to initiate vomiting. The word "bulbar" can also refer to the nerves and tracts connected to the medulla, important in proper swallowing.

Alzheimer's write-up of this patient, posthumously edited and published by Spielmeyer, was titled with reference to the symptoms: "On a Peculiar Disease of the Central Nervous System with Bulbar Symptoms and Painful Spastic Cramps of the Extremities." It appeared in *Zeitschrift fur die Gesamte Neurologie und Psychiatrie*. The word "peculiar" in this title is reminiscent of its similar use by Alzheimer for Deter's Alzheimer's disease:

> All in all we have to face a peculiar disease process. Such peculiar disease processes have been verified recently in considerable numbers.[2]

But how "peculiar" was either case?

This twenty-seven-year old governess was originally admitted to a TB sanatorium. Alzheimer knew his patient was running symptoms of bulbar palsy, which can include progressive difficulty with chewing, talking, and swallowing. Yet eight years before Alzheimer saw this patient, in 1905, Dr. D. J. McCarthy of Phipps Institute at Johns Hopkins described a similar case of bulbar palsy from cerebral tuberculosis, also with difficulty of swallowing, the same brief remission, the same weakness of the arms and legs, and the same fatal termination that Alzheimer's patient would soon experience. Accompanying this, mentioned McCarthy, "Not a cell in the spinal cord was in a normal healthy condition."[3] It has long been known that severe tuberculous meningitis can, in certain cases, produce the same bulbar palsy that Alzheimer's patient had,[4] either through blood-borne seeding or extension from the base of the brain downward to the medulla on its path to the spine.

The medulla is continuous with the spinal cord, which explains Alzheimer's patients' spinally related "painful spastic convulsive states of the extremities."

What is surprising is that this and other cases of CNS spinal involvement with or without TB meningitis were extraordinarily and widely documented in the literature both prior to and during Alzheimer's time. Kelynack,[5] a UK neurologist, mentioned in 1908—just five years before Alzheimer saw his patient—that when cerebral tuberculosis affects the spinal membranes, symptoms in the cervical region could include violent painful contractions in the arm, forearm, and shoulders, usually accompanied by weakness. And lower down, in the lumbar spine region, inflammation from the disease could yield similar painful convulsions and weakness of the lower extremities, creating a stiffness of gait.

By all indications, this young woman was seriously sick and suffering from a systemic/neurological disease with general as well as neurologic symptoms. Yet when Alzheimer turned the case over for presentation to the Breslau Psychiatric–Neurologic

Union in February of 1913, he weighed in with the awkward, if not reckless, conclusion that this young lady was suffering from a hysterical condition of the mind, as first popularized by Sigmund Freud. Alzheimer noted, "An organic disease [such as neurotuberculosis] is unimaginable. Clinical observation points to a strong psychogenic [originating in the mind] suggestibility."[6]

She simply was, then, according to Alzheimer, an open and shut case of psychiatric hysteria.

Dr. Ludwig Mann, extremely familiar with the case, did not agree. To Mann there was no question that the patient had chronic central nervous system disease, and he considered the hysterical symptoms a mere by-product of such disease. Mann could not have been more correct. Within four months of that presentation, this twenty-seven-year-old had seizures, ran a temperature of 41.8 degrees Celsius (107.24 Fahrenheit), became almost entirely unresponsive, and died. Obviously, then, this was a case of more than psychiatric hysteria, and it was time for some damage control. Alzheimer, after the girl's death, made this statement:

> Even if there could now be no doubt that an organic condition lay at the basis of the clinical picture [which there was no longer any doubt], it still appeared quite impossible to classify it with any known illness.[6]

Alzheimer's use of the term "impossible to classify it with any known illness" again sounds like his impression of Auguste Deter with her "Alzheimer's disease." Yet, at least in the case of the deceased twenty-seven-year-old, this statement proves to be presumptive. In the meantime, no serious effort, as with Deter,

was exerted to perform a spinal tap or other diagnostics to rule
out tubercular or other infectious disease.

Alzheimer then admitted what should have been his opening
assessment to begin with:

> Our anatomic and physiological knowledge [of this
> case of the twenty-seven-year old] is burdened with
> countless gaps, which can for this reason easily lead
> us to erroneous conclusions.[6]

Such as jumping to the conclusion that this case was one of
hysteria.

Yet when left with the grizzly task of autopsying this girl,
Alzheimer's findings show serious pathology entirely unre-
lated to a mental condition. At one point, Alzheimer considered
Wilson's disease (hepatolenticular degeneration) in his differential diagnosis. Wilson's disease is thought to be a genetic, cop-
per-hoarding disease, but it should also be noted that acid-fast
forms can cause chromosomal damage and genetic changes.[7]

Although Alzheimer was unable to isolate any organisms during an autopsy from his patient, the stains he used and which
microbes he was looking for were not clearly listed. Yet it was
in Wilson's disease that Dr. Virginia Livingston and Dr. Eleanor
Alexander-Jackson later would isolate acid-fast mycobacterial, tubercular-like microorganisms. Traditionally, since Koch
(1882), mycobacteria such as tuberculosis and leprosy were
identified by their capacity to retain certain red dyes such as
carbol-fuschsin after being rinsed with acid alcohol, a common

laboratory reagent. These microorganisms were and still are therefore called "acid fast."

One of Livingston's cases of Wilson's disease involved a thirty-four-year-old woman. Livingston and Jackson found intracellular acid-fast microorganisms in mice and guinea pigs after injecting them with the bacteria isolated from this woman's blood. These animals then developed the same chronic disease of the liver, spleen, and brain that Livingston's patient had.[8] It is practically medical dictum that any Parkinson's patient under forty should be carefully checked for Wilson's disease.[9] A similar microorganism was cultured from the blood of meningoencephalitis patients by C. G. Burn[10] at the Rockefeller Institute Hospital in New York. But when, in 1970, Livingston and Jackson revisited Burns bacillus,[11] they determined that it, too, stained "acid-fast."

Schömberg, like Breslau, is a town in Silesia, a spa town in the north of the Black Forest in Baden-Württemberg. Breslau sat only fifty-one miles west by southwest of where Alzheimer's Breslau clinic was. By 1911, Dr. Bruno Bandelier, medical director of Schömberg's Schwarswaldheim TB sanatorium, published *A Clinical System of Tuberculosis Describing All Forms of the Disease.*[12] The book, quickly picked up by William Wood and Company in New York, was also readily available to Alois Alzheimer in its original German version by 1911—a year and a half before he saw the ill-fated twenty-seven-year-old governess.

von Fieandt, H. Beitrage zur Kenntniss der Pathogenese und Histologicder experimentellen Meningeal- und Gehirntuberculose, Arbeiten ausdem patholog. Institut der Universitat Helsingfors (Finland). III.235, 1911 (Karger, Berlin).

Bruns, L. Die Geschwülste des Nervensystems, Berlin, 1908.

Veraguth, O., and Bruns, H.Case 1. "Subpialer, makrosopisch intramedullarer Solitartuberkel in der Hohe des vierten und funften cervical segments : Operation." Genesung, Cor.-Bl. f. Schweiz, Aerzte, 1910, XI, 1097; 1147.

Zunker, Tuberkel in der grauen Substanz der Lendenanschwellung, mit Verlust der Schmerzempfindung, Zeit. f. Klin. Med., I, 1880, 375.

de Jonge, Dr. Tumor der Medulla Oblongata ; Diabetes Mellitus. Arch f. Psych u. Nerv., XIII, 1882, 658.

Marfan, Tubercle Solitaire de la Moelle, siegant, au niveau des deuxibme et troisieme paires sacrees. Semaine Medicale, XVII, 189J, 92.

Aniel Robot, Tubercule Primitif de la Moelle; Meningite Tuberculeuse Secondare, Tuberculose, Concomitante des Ganglions Bronchiques de la Pleure, du Poumon, du Foie, de la Rate et du Rein Droit. Lyon Medical, LXXXVIII, 1898, 605.

Gouraud, F. Tubercule de la Moelle Epiniere, Bull. Soc. Anat. de Paris. 1902.

Hunter, W. K. " Case of Tubercular Tumour of the Spinal Cord in a Child Two Years Old." Brain, XXV, 1902, 226.

Luce, Ueber Tuberkulose des Zentralnervensystems (Case reported before the Biologische Abtheilung des drztlichen Vereins, Hamburg, Feb. 17, 1908), Munch. med. Woch., 1908.

Kositz, Ueber Rückenmarkstumoren int Kindesaiter. Wien med. Blatter, 1885, Nr. 42, 1274.

Gerhardt, C. Zwei Falle von Ruckenmarksgeschwulsten, Charite-Annulen, XX. 1893. 162.

Obolonsky, Ueber einen Fall von Reuckenmarkstuberculose mit Verbreitung des tuberculosen Processes auf dem Wege des Centralcanales, Zeit. f. Heilkunde, IX, 1888, 411.

Schiff, Arthur, Ueber zwei Falls von intramedillaren Rückenmarkstumoren, Obersteiner's Arbeiten aus dem Institut für Anatomie und Physiologie, 2, 1894, 155. Intramedullares Tuberkel des Rückenmarks.

Sudek, P. Ein Fall von Tuberkelbildung im Rückenmark, Jahrbilcher der Hamburgschen Staatskrankenanstalten, Bd. IV, 1893-4, 58.

Chvostek, Zwei Fälle von Tuberkulose des Rückenmarkes, Wien. med. Presse, XIV, 1873, 810.

Mueller, L. R. Ueber einen Fall von Tuberculose des Rückenmarkes in it besonderer Berücksichtigung der secunddren Degenerationen, Deutsch. Zeit. f. Nerv., X, 1896-7, 273.

Oberndortfer, Ernest. Ein Fall von Rückenmarkstuberkel, Munch. med. Woch., LI. 1904, 108.

Schultz, Friedrich. Zur Symptomatologie und pathologischen Anatomie der Tuberculosen und entsündlicher Erkrankungen mid der Tuberkel des cerebrospinalen Nervensystems, Dent. Arch. f. klin. Med., XXV, 1880, 297.

Schlesinger, Herman. Ueber Zentrale Tuberculose des Rückenmarkes, Deutsch. Zeit. f. Nerv., VIII, 1895-6, 398.

Mader, Ein Fall von Tuberkulose des Halsmarkes, Wiener, medicinische Presse, XX, 1879, 1056.

Serre, Observations et reflexions sur l'etat de nos connaissances a l'egard de quelques lesions organiques, Gas. Med. de Paris, 1830, Tome, No. 7, 57.

Eisenschitz, J. Tuberkel des Rückenmarks, Jahrb. für Kinderheilkunde, 1870, 224.

Jolly, Ueber tuberkulose Rückenmarkserkrankungen (Report of case before the Gesellschaft der Charite-Aerzte in Berlin), Muenchener medisinische Wocdienschrift, vol. 49, 1902, p. 2026.

Rystedt, G. Ueber einen Fall von Solitartuberkel im Rückenmark mit Nebenbefund von sogenannter artifizieller Heterotopie desselben, Zeit. F klin. Med. LXIII, 1907, 220.

Thorel, Ch. Grosser Solitartuberkel des Ruckenmarks, Deut. med. Woch. XXXIII. 1907, 216. Demonstration of specimen before Aerztlicher Verein in Nurnberg. Nov. 21, 1907.

Mohr, R. Ueber einen Fall von Tuberkulosa des Lendenmarks, Verhand. d. Deutsch. Path. Gesellschaft, Zentral Bd. f. alla. path. Anat., 1909.

Doerr, Carl. Zur Kenntnis der Tuberkulose des Ruckenmarks, Arch.f. Psych. IL, 1911-12, 406.

Lionville, Nouveaux exemples de lesions tuberculeuses dans la moelle epiniere, Arch. gen de med. I, 1875, 92.

Figure 38. A small fraction of the literature directly pertinent to the signs and symptoms of the twenty-seven-year-old governess's case— readily available to Dr. Alzheimer. Such citations regard tubercular involvement of the brain and spinal column. An exponentially greater number of references were in existence at that time.

Bandelier wrote with physician Otto Roepke, at the time director of another German TB sanatorium at Stadwald in Melsungen, near Cassel. It is doubtful whether Alzheimer ever reviewed Bandelier and Roepke's *Die Klinik Der Tuberkulose* or the hundreds and hundreds of well-documented references behind it, but by May 1912, obviously many in the German medical profession had. It required a second edition after only a year and a half and had become a virtual necessity for the medical profession. Its goal: to stimulate further interest in the clinical and practical recognition and treatment of the disease.

Bandelier and Roepke's English version[13] was cited in the March 13, 1913, issue of *Nature*[14] right along with Professors Alzheimer and Nissl's *Histological and Histopathological Work over the Cerebral Cortex*. That Roepke and Bandelier would question Alzheimer's differential diagnosis in the case of the twenty-seven-year-old governess was a given. Besides the multitude of individual signs and symptoms Alzheimer listed that were compatible with tuberculosis of the nervous system, the authors had made this caution:

> Hysteria and tuberculosis approach each other closely. Even a slight tubercular infection, and still more fever, anemia, and inanition may in latent hysteria call forth such severe manifestations that the symptoms of tuberculosis may be masked by those of hysteria; such a condition has been called "hysterical tuberculosis."[13, p. 431]

In no way could Otto Roepke agree with Alzheimer's diagnosis of the twenty-seven-year-old. Alzheimer's charting of "weakness" could quite conceivably have been from an anemia of a chronic disease such as tuberculosis, while *inanition*—lack of mental or spiritual vigor and enthusiasm—often comes across as depression. The symptom of "painful spastic convulsive states of the extremities" speaks for a spinal-cord involvement or compression from the disease, whereas the bulbar symptoms speaks of involvement of the medulla.

———————————

Alzheimer died at only fifty-one, for reasons to this day not certain, but no one at any time has ever said that being a pathologist or neuropathologist was the safest of occupations. Historians report that Alzheimer's encounter with death began with a severe cold with flu-like symptoms, but that infectious endocarditis was responsible for his death.

As early as 1911, Bruno Bandelair and Otto Roepke published their book, in German, in which all of the postmortem explanations for Alzheimer's early death ("infectious angina," infectious endocarditis, nephritic kidney disease, and inflammatory disease of the joints) could be found to spring forth under the umbrella of blood-borne tuberculosis. So the question presents, could Alzheimer have been one of the seven million people worldwide whom TB killed each year at that time?

Infectious endocarditis is no stranger to systemic tuberculosis, as B. C. Millar[15] points out. But even before that, TB, a disease capable of infecting every organ in the body—the heart no exception—was first reported to cause a tuberculous endocarditis (TBE) in 1892[16] and many other cases since. British pathologist/

researcher William Stark [Stark, 1765], explained how, after a flulike lung involvement, TB could and was carried by the bloodstream to various parts of the body, including the heart, the kidney, the joints, and the brain. It could then either turn into progressive disease or reactivate, even decades later. These were the "little lumps" that Stark uncovered on autopsy after autopsy. Pathologist Stark died at age thirty. Stark thus anticipated the tubercular findings of the famed Laennec, a contemporary of Parkinson. But after his death, Stark's words fell on deaf ears, only to become a curious controversy among students in various countries throughout Europe. Among these students was Bichat (1771–1882), a French pathologist who had autopsied countless tuberculous patients before he died of the disease at thirty-one, uttering as follows:

> Not much is really known about the pathology of phthisis [tuberculosis], for few autopsies have been done because of the foolish fear among physicians that the disease is catching.[17]

Both his own untimely death and the findings of Robert Koch would soon prove him wrong.

Just before Bichat died, seasoned pathologist Gaspard Laurent Bayle, also from France, predicted that tuberculosis was an infectious disease before this was proven. He was also first to describe the millet-like seed bodies as "tubercles." Bayle himself died at the age of forty-two. But it was Bayle's junior collaborator, René Laënnec, whom Parkinson personally knew, who would indelibly stamp on the Western mind that not only was tuberculosis infectious, but that it could literally attack every tissue of the human body. Laënnec did hundreds of postmortem examinations of persons who had died of tuberculosis; he died at the age of forty-five.

Not all that much time had elapsed since Alzheimer's discovery of Alzheimer's disease when Neurologist I. J. Sands[18] gave his talk on senile and presenile psychoses for a 1918 clinical conference at Columbia's Department of Neurology in New York City.

After a review of the age-related dementia literature, including that of Alzheimer and Fischer, Sands got around to his own work. Using Alzheimer's own descriptions of the tangles, plaque, and clinical progressive memory loss for a man in his forties, Sands matched Alzheimer with a case that he mentions typified Alzheimer's cases.

Sands first saw this patient, E. K., in late September 1917, and this patient died about a month afterward, three months after admission. Autopsy showed many of the changes typifying Alzheimer's age-related dementia, including a brain very much smaller than normal, definite temporal lobe atrophy, dilated ventricles, and an atrophic cortex. Microscopic findings included a somewhat thickened pia and a definite loss of cells in the first three layers of the cortex. There also was an increase in neuroglia, the presence of senile plaque, and whorls and the snarls of classic tangles.

But there was more. Just across from the bronchopneumonia, on the top of the right lung sat an area of tubercular involvement.

And although Sands, relying on gross findings at autopsy, never did the exhaustive, painstaking slices and stains needed to rule out tubercular central-nervous-system involvement, he nevertheless realized that the disease had spread from the lungs through the blood to other organs because this patient's liver and spleen were also riddled with miliary TB. A gross autopsy nevertheless showed marked atrophy of the cerebrum, the beginning of plaque formation, and neurofibrillary changes. So Sands completed his summary of findings as marked cerebral atrophy, with plaques and tangles of the Alzheimer's type alongside chronic pulmonary tuberculosis of the lungs, liver, and spleen—a scenario not unlike what Southard, Schwartz, and Clouston repeatedly had reported.

NOTES

1. A. Alzheimer, "Uber Eine Eigenartige Erkrankung des Zentralen Nervensystems Mit Bulbaen Symptomen und Schmerzhaften Spastischen Krampfzustanden der Extremitaen," *Zeitschrift fur die Gesamte Neurologie und Psychiatrie* 33 (1916): 45–59.

2. K. Maurer, S. Volk, and H. Gerbaldo, "Auguste D and Alzheimer's Disease," *The Lancet* 349, no. 9064 (May 1997): 1546–9.

3. S. E. Jelliffe, "Proceedings: National Association for the Study and Prevention of Tuberculosis," *The Medical News* 86 (January–June 1905): 1150.

4. F. Gerstenbrand, K. Jellinger, E. Maida, A. Pilz, F. Sandhofer, and G. Weissenbacher, "Symptomatology of the Most Severe Form of Tuberculous Meningitis," *Journal of Neurology* 222, no. 3 (1980): 191–204.

5. T. N. Kelynack, *Tuberculosis in Infancy and Childhood* (London: Bailliere, Tindall, and Cox, 1908).

6. K. Maurer and U. Mauer, *Alzheimer's Disease: The Llife of a Physician and the Career of a Disease* (Chichester, West Sussex: Columbia University Press, 2003), 196.

7. "Department of Anatomy, St. John's Medical College, Bangalore, India," *Tubercle* 71, no. 3 (September 1990):169–72, www.ncbi.nom.nih.gov/pubmed/2238121.

8. V. Wuerthele-Caspe, E. Alexander-Jackson, M. Gregory, L. W. Smith, I. C. Diller, and Z. Mankowski, "Intracellular Acid-Fast Microorganism: Isolated from Two Cases of Hepatolenticular Degeneration," *Journal of the American Medical Women's Association* 11, no. 4 (1956): 120–9.

9. J. Jancovic and E. Tolosa, *Parkinson's Disease and Movement Disorders* (Baltimore: Williams & Wilkins, 1998).

10. C. G. Burn, "Unidentified Gram-Positive Bacillus Associated with Meningo-Encephalitis," *Proceedings of the Society for Experimental Biology and Medicine* 31 (1934): 1095.
11. V. Livingston, "A Specific Type of Organism Cultivated from Malignancy: Bacterial and Proposed Classification," *Annals of the New York Academy of Sciences* 174 (1970): 636–54.
12. ü. Bandelier and Dr. Roepke, *Lehrbuch der Spezifischen Diagnostic und Therapie der Tuberkulose: fur arzte und Studierende* (Wurzburg: Curt Kabitzsch, 1911).
13. B. Bandelier and O. Roepke, *A Clinical System of Tuberculosis*, translated from the Second German Edition by G. Band and Bertram Hunt, MD (New York: William Wood and Company, 1913).
14. "Forthcoming Books," *Nature* 91 (March 13, 1913): 44.
15. B. C. Millar and J. E. Moore, "Emerging Issues in Infective Endocarditis," *Emerging Infectious Diseases* 10, no. 6 (June 2004): 1110–6.
16. A. Liu, E. Nicol, Y. Hu, and A. Coates A, "Tuberculous Endocarditis," *International Journal of Cardiology* 167, no. 3 (August 10, 2013): 640–5.
17. B. L. Gordon, *Ocular Tuberculosis, Its Relation to General Tuberculosis—Ophthalmologic Reviews*, edited by Francis Heed Adler (1944): 541–56.
18. I. J. Sands, "Senile and Presenile Psychosis," *Neurological Bulletin* 1, no. 10 (October 1918): 377–385.

ABOUT THE AUTHOR

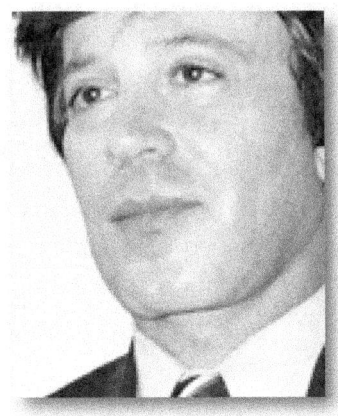

Lawrence Broxmeyer, MD, is a Pennsylvania internist and medical researcher. He was on staff at New York affiliate hospitals of SUNY Downstate, Cornell University, and New York University for approximately fourteen years, part of which was during the height of the US coastal AIDS epidemic.

In conjunction with colleagues in San Francisco and at the University of Nebraska, he pursued, as lead author and originator, a novel technique to kill AIDS mycobacteria and tuberculosis, producing outstanding results (see the *Journal of Infectious Diseases*, October 15, 2002: 186(8): 1155–60). His ideas on killing intracellular pathogens by phage have influenced and stimulated further research in this area.

Recently he contributed a chapter regarding these findings to Sleator and Hill's textbook *Patho-Biotechnology*, published by Landes Bioscience. In addition, Broxmeyer has written many peer-reviewed articles, available on PubMed of the US Library of Medicine, National Institutes of Health, at http://www.ncbi.nlm.nih.gov/pubmed?term=broxmeyer%20L.

Broxmeyer's research covers the most challenging medical problems of our times, including AIDS, Alzheimer's disease, diabetes, Parkinson's, and cardiovascular disease. Among the books that Broxmeyer has published are *Parkinson's—Another Look* by New Century Press, now in its third edition, and *AIDS: What the Discoverers of HIV Have Never Admitted.*

INDEX